HAVING A FIRST BABY:
EXPERIENCES IN 1951 AND 1985 COMPARED

Having a First Baby Experiences in 1951 and 1985 Compared

Two social, obstetric and dietary studies of married primigravidae in Aberdeen

Barbara Thompson
Cynthia Fraser
Angela Hewitt
Debbie Skipper

ABERDEEN UNIVERSITY PRESS

First Published 1989
Aberdeen University Press
A Member of the Pergamon Group

© Barbara Thompson, Cynthia Fraser, Angela Hewitt and Debbie Skipper 1989

British Library Cataloguing in Publication Data

Having a first baby: experiences in 1951
    and 1985 compared: two social, obstetric
    and dietry studies of married primigravidae
    in Aberdeen
    1. Women. Pregnancy & childbirth.
    Sociological perspectives
    I. Thompson, Barbara
    306.8′743

ISBN 0 08 036596 5

Printed in Great Britain
The University Press
Aberdeen

Foreword

The research reported in this monograph was inspired by the late Professor Sir Dugald Baird who was Regius Professor of Obstetrics and Gynaecology in the University of Aberdeen from 1937 until his retirement in 1965.

His experience as a medical student attending home confinements of women in the Glasgow slums in the 1920s was fundamental to shaping his career. Throughout his life he vividly recalled the appalling living conditions, the fatalism of mothers old beyond their years, the high maternal and infant mortality and the apathetic and rachitic children. Later he also became aware of the wide variations in the health and reproductive efficiency between women in private and in hospital practice. He once said, 'The contrast between childbearing in the upper social classes and in the slum dweller set me thinking about social class differences in the whole field of reproduction and so my lasting interest in social research in the field of obstetrics began.'

By moving to Aberdeen, Sir Dugald saw unrivalled opportunities for the research he believed to be necessary in order to establish the facts and to fulfill what he considered was the role of the obstetrician in society (Baird, 1971). The Aberdeen population was of an appropriate size and of a settled nature which would allow follow-up of women and their families, and there was a centralised medical service. The war delayed his plans, but he set about establishing a record system based on good quality data and accurate measurements as the basis for epidemiological analysis. After the introduction of the National Health Service he gave up private practice to concentrate on research.

Before he came to Aberdeen Sir Dugald had gained academic distinction and earned a reputation as an original thinker and fearless scientific investigator. In the late 1940s he took the unprecedented and controversial step of introducing an epidemiologist, a physiologist, psychologist, and statistician as well as dietitians and sociologists to his department. Such actions aroused some hostility in a reactionary profession, but he was able to persuade the Medical Research Council to support such interdisciplinary research within the London based Social Medicine Research Unit (Professor J N Morris) until in 1955 the Obstetric Medicine Research Unit was established in Aberdeen with Sir Dugald as honorary director. This was disbanded when he retired, but the sociological team formed the nucleus of a new MRC Medical Sociology Unit (Professor R Illsley) to which Sir Dugald remained attached until he moved to Edinburgh in 1978 where he continued to produce scientific papers containing original data (for example, Baird, 1985) until his death in 1986.

During the 1940s, Sir Dugald published numerous papers on social class differences in childbearing and on nutrition (for example, Baird, 1945; 1946; 1947; 1948; 1949).

Towards the end of the decade, ably assisted by Dr Angus M Thomson, he initiated a wide range of co-ordinated epidemiological studies: the results of these led to greater understanding of factors affecting childbearing and influenced clinical practice. This pioneer work carried out in Aberdeen was highly influential when the 1958 British Perinatal Mortality Survey (Butler and Bonham, 1963; Butler and Alberman, 1969) was being designed. The success of the early research in Aberdeen resulted from there being a clear objective, i.e. making childbearing a safe and as far as possible a pleasant experience for women with the outcome a good sized, normal and healthy baby and with successful breast feeding. To this end scientific methods were applied in answering well designed and specific questions, but potential explanations for certain findings were also sought in the social sciences (Baird, 1949). Some of the early research will be referred to in the course of this monograph, but a brief illustration of the ramifications is given here.

Sir Dugald's initial concern was focused on stillbirths and early deaths (Baird, 1947) which at that time were often referred to as 'obstetric deaths'. This term he used to challenge obstetricians, asserting that some of these deaths might be prevented by different management. Factors associated with such deaths were analysed and causes determined as far as possible (Duncan et al., 1952; Baird et al., 1953; 1954). Postmaturity was a factor and further studies showed that this was associated with fetal anoxia (Walker and Turnbull, 1953) and, therefore, a policy of induction was decided. Short stature was another factor associated with long labour. Studies of height and pelvic shape showed that some men and women brought up in conditions of poverty had a mis-shapen pelvis (Bernard, 1952) which in women could lead to difficulty in labour: the height below which this might occur was established and a policy of booking and elective Caesarean section agreed (Baird, 1955). Another factor was high blood pressure and detailed studies led to definitions of grades of pre-eclampsia and hypertension (Nelson, 1955) with implications for management, which are still used today: generational and familial studies of pre-eclampsia were also undertaken (Adams and Finlayson, 1961). And so, research developed, always based on first hand data for a total population of a geographical area (Chapter 1) with the effect of any innovations carefully assessed (for example, Baird, 1963; Baird et al., 1968).

Parallel to these obstetric orientated studies were others which considered behaviour in pregnancy and labour in relation to intelligence test scores and attitudes to maternity (Scott, 1954; Scott et al., 1956a and b; Scott and Thomson, 1956a and b) and to personality in cases of difficult labour (Stewart and Scott, 1953; Cramond, 1954) Sociologists were also asking questions such as the effect of paid work during pregnancy (Illsley et al.,

1954). More importantly, however, they were studying various aspects of selection, e.g. in-migration (Illsley *et al.*, 1963) and marriage (Thompson, 1956) and helping to explain why differences between social classes remained, e.g. a high neonatal and infant mortality in the lower social classes, in spite of a marked overall fall over decades (Titmuss, 1943). In major research Illsley (1955: 1956*a*) studied the factors which led to social differentiation between occupational groups and the mechanisms which linked health to occupational status. He showed how the process of social mobility produced a tendency to perpetuate disparity.

It became obvious that reproductive efficiency depended on long-term social influences which were related to physical growth, development and health. Thus, the focus turned to generational considerations and Sir Dugald with American collaborators (Birch *et al.*, 1970) made the first known study of the influence of mothers' experience of pregnancy and delivery on the mental and physical development of children from birth into adolescence.

Sir Dugald's approach was much broader than that adopted by the survey reported in Maternity in Great Britain (Douglas, 1948) which took the view that reproductive performance was greatly affected by social influences acting during the nine months of pregnancy as well as by the organisation of the maternity services. As Sir Dugald said:

> The mother's ability to play her part depends on *the quality of her own environment in utero and from birth till she reaches maturity*. Hereditary factors also play a part, but are not well understood yet. The standard of care depends on the quality of the training of doctors and midwives, the efficiency of the organisation of medical and nursing services, and their availability to the public. This depends to a large extent on how much money the community is prepared to spend on medical services. (Baird, 1969)

Sir Dugald was a great champion of the interests of women's health and of their right to choose on the question of fertility which he saw as fundamentally important not only to the individual, but to the well-being of her family, and ultimately to that of society as a whole. To this end he played a major part in revolutionising the pattern of human reproduction, not only in North-East Scotland, but in Britain. He focused on what he called 'A Fifth Freedom?', adding to the four freedoms defined by Franklin Roosevelt another, namely that women 'should be free from the tyranny of excessive fertility' (Baird, 1965). In partnership with the local health authority he ensured that family planning services were available to all Aberdeen women. He also began offering abortion to women for social reasons. Aberdeen experience played an important part in the evolution of abortion law reform culminating in the Abortion Act 1967. He also encouraged women who wanted to be finished with childbearing to consider sterilisation, and in conjunction with the Simon Population Trust persuaded surgeons to carry out the first vasectomies in Aberdeen. He saw deaths from cervical cancer as unnecessary tragedies usually affecting young families (Aitken-Swan and Baird, 1965; 1966) and he initiated the first screening service for a total population in Britain, providing a model for other areas (Macgregor and Baird, 1963).

The Department built up an international reputation as publications on reproductive epidemiology, physiology, endocrinology and medical sociology proliferated. Sir Dugald gained international renown and travelled extensively. Wherever he went he applied the epidemiological approach he had adopted in Aberdeen to checking his 'hunches' about childbearing, whether in sophisticated teaching hospitals or isolated villages in developing countries. On my return from secondment to conduct a socio-medical study of marriage, childbirth and early childhood in an isolated African village, he handed me several files of detailed raw data he had personally collected or copied from medical records and partially analysed during visits to Hong Kong, North Borneo, Sarawak and Western Nigeria: these served as additional tropical data for comparison with Aberdeen in trying to identify patterns and 'natural laws' of childbearing (Thompson and Baird, 1967).

He was knighted in 1959 and received many honours, including honorary degrees from numerous universities. In 1966 he and his wife (the late May Tennent, who had been Chairman of the North-East Regional Hospital Board) made local history, when in a joint ceremony, they were both given the Freedom of the City of Aberdeen.

Sir Dugald's breadth of vision, energy and dedication to his objectives were remarkable and much of what he pioneered, revolutionary at the time, is now generally accepted practice. He inspired people wherever he went and encouraged rigorous standards in research. His influence is incalculable and is disseminated by at least 25 of his staff who became professors in Britain and abroad. He was an outstanding leader and teacher, a man of great character, with the courage of his own convictions, who was also distinguished for his friendliness, compassion and interest in people as individuals.

Personally, I am deeply indebted to Sir Dugald for the opportunities he provided and for his unfailing encouragement to me throughout my career. Regrettably, he died before the results of the research reported in this monograph were available, otherwise his erudite comments would undoubtedly have enhanced the discussion.

Barbara Thompson

Contents

List of Tables and Figures

FIGURES

Abbreviations

AMH	Aberdeen Maternity Hospital
ANC	Antenatal Clinic
APH	Antepartum haemorrhage
ARM	Artificial rupture of membranes
BF	Breast Feeding
CHO	Carbohydrate
CS	Caesarean section
D&C	Dilatation and curettage
ECG	Electrocardiograph
FPC	Family Planning Clinic
GP	General practitioner
IUCD	Intrauterine contraceptive device
LBW	Low birthweight—less than 2,500g
LMP	Last menstrual period
MRC	Medical Research Council
NCT	National Childbirth Trust
NHS	National Health Service
NS	Not statistically significant
PE	Pre-eclampsia
PMR	Perinatal mortality rate
PNC	Prenuptial conception—marriage during pregnancy
PNM	Perinatal mortality
PPH	Postpartum haemorrhage
RGIT	Robert Gordon's Institute of Technology, Aberdeen
TB	Tuberculosis
t	'Student' t test not paired
$\lambda_{(i)}^2$	Suffix = degrees of freedom

Acknowledgements

We would like to thank the many people, who, in so many different ways, facilitated the conduct of this research. The 1984–5 study could not have been undertaken without the co-operation of Professor Ian MacGillivray and the obstetricians. The primigravidae attended the antenatal clinics conducted by Professor MacGillivray and Dr Doris M Campbell, to whom we are especially grateful for their support and help throughout the project. Also we thank Mrs M Bramley and the antenatal clinic staff for making the necessary arrangements and providing accommodation for the interviewing. We thank Mrs Heather Dietz, research dietitian, who was conducting diet surveys for a vitamin study, for her co-operation when the two studies overlapped. We are also grateful to Miss Kathleen Ross for general advice on the diet survey.

We acknowledge with gratitude the advice and help which we received from Mr John Lemon in computing and processing the social and obstetric data. Mrs Gillian Lockie and Dr A Wise gave initial advice and kindly provided the computer programme used in calculating the 1984–85 dietary intakes. We are indebted to Mr David Hunter for his invaluable help in computing and analysing the dietary data. The comparison with the 1950–51 diet survey could not have been made without the co-operation of Professor A M Thomson, who provided the Cope-chat cards from which the data were extracted, he was helpful throughout and commented on the results. Miss Jean Marr, MBE answered some queries on the earlier diet survey and on food rationing at that time. Dr E M Fotheringham confirmed details of the psychological enquiry and the overlap with the social and dietary studies.

In the preparation of this report, Mr M Samphier provided the background epidemiological data for Chapter 2, and the Department of Medical Illustrations produced all the Figures. We gratefully acknowledge comments received on the draft of this monograph from Miss J Aitken-Swan, MBE, Dr D M Campbell, Mrs A Finlayson, Dr M H Hall, Dr D Lloyd, Professor I MacGillivray, Dr S Macintyre, Dr I Russell and Professor A A Templeton. We also thank Mrs I Morrison for the final typing.

Our special thanks go to the mothers in Aberdeen who co-operated in both studies and who generously gave of their time and welcomed us into their homes.

Authors

CYNTHIA FRASER, MA, Dip Ed (Aberdeen) is a psychologist who previously undertook the testing and assessment of children in a study of low birthweight. She has also reviewed the literature on selected perinatal procedures for the World Health Organisation. In the research reported in this monograph she was responsible for computing the data and the analysis as well as sharing the interviewing of the 1984-5 sample. She is now on the staff of the Department of Obstetrics and Gynaecology, University of Aberdeen.

ANGELA HEWITT, MA (Aberdeen) was previously the Organiser and Administrative Officer for a study of low birthweight and later prepared background reports on three areas in Scotland relating to research on policy and the provision of social services. On the 1984-5 project she shared the interviewing and acted as administrative officer and secretary.

DEBBIE SKIPPER, Dip Dietetics (RGIT, Aberdeen) was previously a research dietitian in the Department of Obstetrics and Gynaecology. She conducted the 1984-5 diet survey.

BARBARA THOMPSON, OBE, BA, Dip Soc Studies (Manchester), PhD (Aberdeen) was involved in the original interdisciplinary study of primigravidae in Aberdeen. In the early 1960s she was seconded to the MRC Laboratories in The Gambia and her PhD thesis was on marriage, childbirth and early childhood in an isolated village. Later she was responsible for the fertility related research carried out in the MRC Medical Sociology Unit. She directed the 1984-5 project, shared the interviewing in both studies and takes responsibility for the results and conclusions reported in this monograph. She was awarded the OBE in 1983. Since she retired in 1986 she has been an Honorary Research Fellow in the Department of Obstetrics and Gynaecology, University of Aberdeen and Honorary Attached Worker to the MRC Medical Sociology Unit in Glasgow.

All the contributors were on the staff of the MRC Medical Sociology Unit in Aberden when the 1984-5 research was carried out.

CHAPTER 1

Background and Method

This monograph reports a comparative study of the social, dietary and obstetric characteristics and behaviour of two samples of married women resident in Aberdeen whose first pregnancy ended in a birth in 1950–1 or in 1984–5.

As stated in the Foreword the earlier study was inspired by the late Professor Sir Dugald Baird and arose out of his enquiries into the incidence and causes of stillbirths in the city of Aberdeen which indicated the importance of the maternal environment (Baird, 1945; 1947; 1949). Recognising the likely significance of diet, in 1948 he launched a survey of the diet of pregnant women in Aberdeen. He soon decided, however, that in order to explain dietary differences it would be necesary to undertake parallel social and psychological studies as he reckoned that any dietary differences between women were most likely to have their origins in different kinds of social experiences, education and customs.

In 1949–50, the research team he appointed, which was partly funded by the Medical Research Council (MRC), included a sociologist, psychologist and social fieldworkers in addition to the existing dietitians and medical staff. After a pilot enquiry, the economic aspects of founding a family were studied in a related but independent research project undertaken within the Department of Political Economy at Aberdeen University (Rowntree, 1954).

One of the authors (BT) took part in the original research and in 1984–5 duplicated the social and dietary enquiry, as far as possible, in order to establish whether associations between social, dietary and obstetric factors identified in 1950–1 were still apparent or whether these had changed. For example, in the early 1950s there was a social class gradient, women in the lower social classes being most likely to be short in stature, native Aberdonians and less well educated; to marry during pregnancy and to attend late for antenatal care; to have poor housing, to eat less protein, to be younger when they had their first babies more of whom were of low birthweight; they were least likely to use contraception, to breast feed and to seek professional advice. In the intervening years there has been a revolution in obstetric technology as well as widespread social changes, including slum clearance, the advent of television, supermarkets, oral contraception, and greater opportunities for education and work. In addition, Aberdeen has experienced the industrial and social impact of North Sea oil exploitation. Given these changes, it is important to consider how they have affected the experiences of primigravidae.

1

The Background in Aberdeen

The interest in the social and preventive aspects of obstetrics developed in the Department of Midwifery (later Obstetrics) and Gynaecology under Sir Dugald Baird and established Aberdeen as the centre for pioneer epidemiological and social obstetric research in the 1950s. The research developed under his Honorary Directorship of the MRC Obstetric Medicine Research Unit until his retirement in 1965 and subsequently continued through the collaboration of the MRC Medical Sociology Unit (Director, Professor Raymond Illsley) with the Department of Obstetrics and Gynaecology (Professor Ian MacGillivray).

Some advantages of Aberdeen for social obstetric research have been as follows:

1. Relative isolation. Although this has been greatly eroded with the development of the oil industry since the early 1970s and by improvements in travel and communications, Aberdeen remains the urban administrative and commercial centre for a large agricultural hinterland, and the educational and medical centre for North East Scotland.

2. Self-sufficient centralised maternity services. In the early 1950s the Aberdeen Maternity Hospital (AMH) and its three associated Homes catered for the vast majority of maternity patients living in the City, the remainder being delivered either in one of three private Nursing Homes under the care of consultant obstetricians or at home by domiciliary midwifes and general practitioners (GPs). However, the private Nursing Homes closed down, one by one, to be replaced by private beds in a wing of AMH. Domiciliary practice virtually disappeared and one of the AMH associated Homes was closed. Throughout the years no Aberdeen obstetrician has been in full-time private practice. Thus, by 1984–5, the maternity services were concentrated on AMH and two associated Homes. In recent years there have been important changes in the provision of antenatal care with more involvement of GPs and a schedule of care based on rational clinical assessment, which is well documented elsewhere (Hall *et al.*, 1980; Chng *et al.*, 1980; Hall *et al.*, 1985). However, in the 1950s and in the 1980s all who wished to be confined in hospital attended a central Antenatal Clinic (ANC) for initial screening and assessment of risk and recommendation for care and booking arrangements.

3. Total population. Initially, research was based on the population of the City of Aberdeen, a compact urban local government area. It was possible to centralise the maternity records for the total city population with the collaboration of the Medical Officer of Health (Dr I A G MacQueen) and the matrons of the private Nursing Homes in conjunction with the obstetricians and general practitioners. However, under the reorganisation of local government in 1975, the Aberdeen City District was created, taking in the City plus populous suburban areas. For maternity research purposes in the 1950s the suburban population was relatively small, but it mushroomed in growth in the 1970s. Thus, although the Aberdeen Maternity and Neonatal Data Bank (Samphier and Thompson, 1981) has been augmented retrospectively to accommodate to this wider area for epidemiological purposes, the 1950–1 study was restricted to women living within the Aberdeen City boundary, whereas that for 1984–5 was based on the Aberdeen City District population. According to the 1951 Census, the usually resident population of the City of Aberdeen was 183,247 and its area was 10,488 acres (General Registry Office, Edinburgh, 1953). The 1981 Census gave the usually resident population of the Aberdeen City District as 199,827 in a much increased land area of roughly 45,582 acres (Registrar General Scotland, 1982).

The Study Population

The original study was based on:

1. Primigravidae—for the following reasons:
(a) Primigravidae are the least selected group of the child bearing population. With pregnancy number or parity, groups become increasingly more selective. Also in order to reduce the variables, only women whose first pregnancies ended in a birth (live or stillbirth) were included, as the management and outcome of a pregnancy might be influenced by a previous pregnancy experience.
(b) Primigravidae present the most frequent obstetric problems, certain conditions being virtually restricted to them.
(c) Primigravidae are more likely to be influenced by their social background as they are relatively young and without parental experience.
(d) A practical consideration was that primigravidae were most likely to have the time and commitment to co-operate. The women were required to invest a good deal of time in undertaking weighed diet and budgetary surveys, psychological tests and interviews with social fieldworkers.

2. Married women only. The study was restricted to women who were married when they first attended the ANC (see Chapter 2). The unmarried, a few of whom married before delivery, were excluded because of their social and obstetric bias and atypical family and personal experiences (Thompson, 1956; Illsley, 1956a). For example, in the 1950s unmarried primigravidae were usually young, lower social class women who attended late, if at all, for antenatal care and delivered an excess of low birthweight babies (less than 2500g).

The Samples

The 1950–1 study was based on a 1 in 6 random sample of married women living in Aberdeen City when they first attended the central ANC during their first pregnancy and booked for confinement in AMH. The same procedure and definitions were adopted in 1984–5 for the Aberdeen City District population, but in order to give adequate numbers in the time available, the random sample was increased to 1 in 4 initially and later to 1 in 3.

1950–1 STUDY

The earlier study was of much wider scope than the later study and went through several phases. The dietary, social and psychological studies started and ended at different times and the method of selection for the diet and social surveys changed.

When the social study began early in 1950, after a pilot investigation, the diet survey had been under way for nearly a year. Parallel studies were then carried out in the 1 in 6 random sample of married primigravidae as defined above Some months later the psychologist joined the team and became responsible for collecting certain new items of information, e.g. use of contraception. The dietitians found, after a time, that they had inadequate numbers of women whose husbands were in professional and managerial or in semi-skilled and unskilled manual occupations, and therefore they

TABLE 1.1
1950–1 RANDOM SAMPLE

Social survey		No. of women
1 in 6 random sample		220
Losses		
Not pregnant	1	
Spontaneous abortion	2	
Not first pregnancy	1	7
Left Aberdeen	3	
Data for analysis		213
Diet survey		
1 in 6 random sample		127*
Losses		
Refused	5	
Data incomplete or unreliable	28	33
Data reliable for analysis		94

* excludes 86 women in the social survey who were not eligible for the diet survey

decided to ask only those women whose husbands were in the Registrar General's social classes I and II, or in IV and V to do a weighed diet survey.

It was estimated that 220 women would be included in the 1984-5 sample, and data on the same number of the 1 in 6 random sample of 1950-1 primigravidae were extracted for comparison. All these women had taken part in the social enquiry, but some were recruited before the psychological study began, while in the later stages only those women whose husbands were in occupations at each end of the social scale, were included in the diet survey (Figure 1.1*).

The data required for these 220 primigravidae had to be collated from a variety of proformas, Cope-Chat Cards and narrative records and processed for computerisation. Included are data on about half the women who took part in the psychological study, but less than half of those who co-operated in the diet and social enquiries, which spanned 1949-55. More comprehensive details of the various aspects of the wider research project are given elsewhere (Illsley, 1956a, Scott, 1954; Thomson, 1958; 1959a and b; Scott and Thomson, 1956a and b; Scott et al., 1956a and b).

In view of the method adopted in the 1950s, the co-operation of the women in the social enquiry was assured and it would have been difficult for them to refuse. However, a few women did not wish to take part in the psychological interviews or to do a diet survey. Also, after selection, several women were lost to the study for other reasons (Table 1.1).

1984-5 STUDY

From the estimated numbers of eligible primigravidae it was decided that in the time available it would be appropriate to recruit a random sample of 1 in 4. However, numbers were less than expected and after a few months the recruitment was increased to 1 in 3. In one year from March 1984, 203 women were recruited, rather fewer than estimated.

The unexpectedly slow recruitment at the beginning of the study meant that in order to obtain the proposed sample size, selection was protracted, and to have included some women recruited towards the end would have meant extending the diet surveys and postnatal visits beyond the time allowed. The timing of the 1984-5 study had to be strictly controlled because of BT's impending retirement, and twelve women recruited to the random sample were excluded.

Other women did not participate in the research for various reasons (Table 1.2). Three women who initially agreed to take part, refused to do the diet survey at the required time, but were willing to be included in the social study.

So data for analysis and comparison are available on 213 women in the 1950-1 study and 158 women in the 1984-5 and also on 94 and 142 reliable weighed diet surveys in the two studies respectively.

* Figures appear at the end of each chapter where appropriate.

TABLE 1.2
1984–5 RANDOM SAMPLE

Social survey		No. of women
Random sample		203
Losses		
Spontaneous abortion	8	
Not first pregnancy	1	
Left Aberdeen	6	
Attended satellite ANC	8	
Refused	10	
Outwith cut-off date	12	45
Data for analysis		158
Diet survey		
Random sample		158
Losses		
Refused	3	
Data incomplete or unreliable	13	16
Data reliable for analysis		142

Method

1950–1 STUDY

The earlier research was conducted as a combined social, psychological and dietary study as shown in Figure 1.1.

1. Recruitment. Every woman who wanted to be confined in hospital attended an ANC located in the city centre. At the first visit she was seen by one of three 'Lady almoners' who were practising case workers and who attended in rotation. These almoners shared all the social fieldwork and recorded a brief social history for every primigravida. Those women who met the criteria were listed in order of attendance and every sixth one was identified for the research project. At the time there was no appointment system and the clinical examination and booking for confinement took place when the woman first attended. All primigravidae were booked for delivery in AMH.

Subsequently, women in the 1 in 6 random sample were requested to co-operate at different stages of pregnancy and postnatally as follows.

2. Psychological tests and interview at 6 months. The women were required to attend the ANC to see the psychologist for two one-hour sessions during which they were asked to complete three psychological tests and assessments were made of their commitment to pregnancy and motherhood and their adjustment to and expectations of marriage (Scott, 1954).

3. Weighed diet survey in 7th month. In the seventh month each woman was seen at the ANC by one of two dietitians and invited to undertake the weighing and recording of her food for one week. If the woman agreed the dietitian arranged to visit her at home and deliver scales and a record book to be used for the survey. The dietitian usually visited again once or twice during the week in order to ensure that the woman knew exactly what was required, was weighing items accurately and was maintaining the record book. At the end of the week the dietitian made a final check and collected the scales and record book. It had been hoped to use these records of menus and weights for re-analysis and descriptive purposes, but regrettably it was found that they had been destroyed and only calculated values of the main dietary intakes are available.

4. Social interview at home in 8th month. At the beginning of the eighth month a social fieldworker visited each woman at home in order to obtain a more detailed social history and knowledge of the social and environmental conditions in which she lived.

5. Postnatal visit at 13 weeks. As the social fieldworkers were attached to AMH where all the mothers were delivered, nearly all mothers were seen when they were admitted for delivery, but their obstetric history was obtained only from medical records. The purpose of the postnatal visit was to collect information about any changes in housing, living arrangements or social circumstances, and about any health problems and the baby's feeding history.

At both the antenatal and the postnatal home visit the fieldworker completed a proforma, which was elaborated by a narrative account dictated subsequently.

Information on contraception used in the present postnatal analysis was obtained five years later when the mother and child attended AMH for a check on the child's health and development.

THE 1984–5 STUDY

The 1984–5 study was constrained by the definitions and limitations of the 1950–1 enquiry, but the opportunity was taken to obtain certain additional information not relevant in 1950–1, e.g. the husband's attendance at the delivery. The recent study had no psychological component and there was a single home visit at thirteen weeks postpartum. It was limited in time and resources not only by the impending retirement of BT, but also by the relocation of the MRC Medical Sociology Unit in Glasgow in 1985.

1. Recruitment. The antenatal arrangements had changed in that all women now attended the central ANC located at AMH by appointment one week before their first medical consultation, in order to be weighed and measured, and to have a blood sample taken and their medical history recorded. At the same time a brief social history was obtained by a research clerkess. From this information married women in their first pregnancy were identified and every fourth (later every third) was told about the research project and invited to participate. For practical purposes it was necessary to restrict the study to primigravidae who received all their antenatal care at the central ANC at AMH. If for any reason a woman particularly wished to attend a satellite clinic this was accepted, and a few women were lost to the study as a result.

2. Diet Survey. It was possible to arrange for the majority of the primigravidae in the study to attend a clinic conducted by Professor Ian MacGillivray and Dr Doris Campbell who, over the years, had carried out metabolic studies involving dietary surveys (e.g. Campbell *et al.*, 1979; 1982). In the course of working with these obstetricians, the dietitian (DS) had helped to validate the method used in conducting the present dietary study (Johnstone *et al.*, 1981). For personal reasons, e.g. wishing to see a particular obstetrician, a few primigravidae attended other clinics at AMH, and special arrangements were made to see them. Also in the later part of the study there was some overlap with a research project on vitamin intake. This required a weighed diet survey at about 30 weeks gestation and by chance eight women were recruited to both projects. By arrangement between the dietitians, one weighed survey was made to serve for both purposes.

In accordance with the redesigned rationalised schedule of antenatal care (Hall *et al.*, 1985), all women were required to attend for clinical examination as near as possible to 30 weeks gestation. In the course of this visit the dietitian saw each primigravida in the random sample and explained what was involved in doing a weighed diet survey for one week. If the woman agreed to take part she was given scales and a record book together with telephone numbers so that she could contact the dietitian at any time if she had any query. She was asked to return the following week and the dietitian then went through the record in detail with her. At this point the dietitian described the social component of the research and if the woman was willing, she was referred on for the social interview.

3. Social interview. The vast majority of these interviews were carried out at the ANC at 31–2 weeks gestation, but six women who had been admitted to AMH were seen in the wards. Information was obtained comparable to that available for the 1950–1 study with certain additional items previously not relevant. In the course of the interview the woman was asked to agree to a postnatal home visit at 13 weeks, and arrangements were made about how to contact her.

Although all the women were admitted for delivery to AMH, for practical reasons the research team were only able to see a minority of them while they were in hospital.

4. Thirteen week postnatal interview.   Once again this visit provided details of changes in the social environment and was also concerned with the woman's health and the baby's feeding and progress. However, in contrast to the 1950-1 study, the women were asked in detail about their delivery and hospital experience for comparison with the medical records.

A precoded proforma was used at both the ANC interview and the postnatal home interview, with space being allowed for the interviewer to comment and to record selected remarks made by the women.

Some factors about the two studies which are indicative of changes in public knowledge, in attitudes and in the social situation may be noted. Before the recent project began it had to be approved in writing by the Senior Obstetric and Gynaecological Staff Committee, to be notified to the Grampian Health Board Joint Ethical Committee, and co-operation had to be obtained from the General Practice Sub-Committee, and from the Community Health Service. In contrast, in 1950-1 the project was not presented as 'research' as at that time there was some trepidation about the connotations of the word and how it might be interpreted. It was only necessary to express the 'interest of Professor Baird' or of 'the Maternity Hospital'. However, as time went on and research developed women increasingly volunteered, particularly after the opening of the Research Unit at AMH which provided a suite of single and double rooms and a day room. One of the attractions of the 1984-5 study to the women participating was that they were booked for delivery in the Research Unit, although eventually a few had to be accommodated in the main wards at AMH if there were no vacant research beds when they were admitted. In conducting the 1950s project most home visits were unannounced as a matter of expediency, whereas in 1984-5 the postnatal home visit was by appointment, facilitated by the fact that nearly all the women were on the telephone, which was fairly rare in the early 1950s.

In the 1950-1 study the three social fieldworkers and two dietitians had to rely on public transport. In 1984-5 two of the fieldworkers had private cars, and the third relied on public transport; the dietitian saw the women only at the ANC at AMH.

RESPONSIBILITY FOR INFORMATION COLLECTED

In the 1950s there was some overlap between the dietitians, the psychologist and the social fieldworkers, e.g. all obtained information on a woman's housing conditions; the psychologist and the social fieldworker independently discussed her family background and occupational history. Thus, any omissions or discrepancies in certain sets of data could usually be clarified by reference to another source, and there was a good deal of cross checking (Illsley, 1956a). However, certain items which had been obtained by the psychologist alone in 1950-1, e.g. family intentions, attitude to breast feeding, and smoking habits were routinely collected in the 1984-5 study.

In the 1984–5 study all the information except that specific to the weighed diet survey and smoking (antenatally) which were dealt with by the dietitian, was obtained at the social interviews. Some additional items were included indicative of social changes, e.g. cohabitation before marriage, and the husband's participation etc., and these will be clearly identified in the analysis.

NOTE

Most of the women who participated in the studies were delivered in the years 1951 and 1985 respectively. For the sake of simplicity, therefore, in what follows the studies will be referred to by these single years only.

FIGURE 1.1   DIAGRAM SHOWING 1950–1 SAMPLE OVERLAP

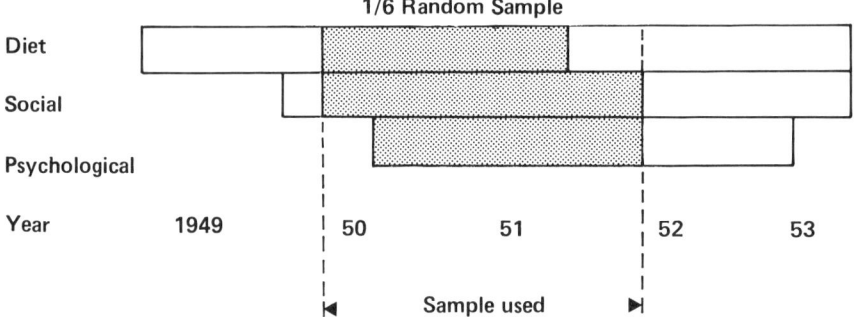

CHAPTER 2

The Relevance of Aberdeen Experience

There are two questions which have to be answered in order to assess whether the Aberdeen studies have any general relevance:

1. How far has Aberdeen's experience over the years followed trends similar to those elsewhere and nationally?
2. How far were the samples of women studied in the early 1950s and mid 1980s representative of the Aberdeen primiparae from whom they came?

1. Overall trends

Figure 2.1 shows the rates of livebirths, stillbirths and neonatal mortality from 1950–85 by three year averages for Aberdeen compared with Dundee, the nearest and most comparable city and with national rates for Scotland and for England and Wales.

Throughout the years, the birth rate in Aberdeen was lower than that for both Dundee and Scotland and also lower than that for England and Wales from the early 1960s. However, atypically there was no marked rise in the Aberdeen birth rate in the late 1950s as occurred elsewhere. This may be accounted for by the readiness of the Aberdeen obstetricians to offer sterilisation as Baird (1965) has described in his well known paper entitled *A Fifth Freedom?* All the birth rates showed a steep decline from the mid 1960s to the late 1970s followed by a rise and then a levelling off except in Dundee where the rise continued (Figure 2.1a).

There was a marked fall in all stillbirth rates (Figure 2.1b). In the 1950s the Aberdeen rate was notably low reflecting actions taken as a result of research undertaken by Baird and his staff in identifying the causes of 'obstetric deaths' and taking policy decisions for prevention (Baird *et al.*, 1953; 1954). As the stillbirth rates declined, Aberdeen lost its early advantage and by 1985 the rates were all at a similar low level.

The pattern of neonatal mortality (Figure 2.1c) is similar to that for stillbirths. Perinatal mortality was not separately defined in the earlier years, but in the last two decades trends have been very similar to those of neonatal mortality, in general Aberdeen having lost its favourable position to Dundee.

Over the years Aberdeen rates for live births, stillbirths and neonatal mortality have been nearer those for England and Wales than those for Scotland and the same applied to Dundee rates in the last two decades. In the earlier years all these rates were higher in Scotland than in England and Wales, but in recent years they have reached similar low levels.

By definition the Aberdeen studies of primigravidae excluded those whose baby was born illegitimate and those whose first pregnancy had ended in abortion whether spontaneous or induced. In Britain an increasing proportion of pregnancies which end in an illegitimate birth are first pregnancies to single women. This also applies to abortions carried out under the Abortion Act 1967, which accounts for the vast majority of first pregnancies which end in abortion. The overall published figures of illegitimacy and induced abortion give some indication of exclusions from the Aberdeen studies.

Figure 2.2a shows that the pattern of live births which were illegitimate in Aberdeen between 1950–85 was similar to that for Scotland and for England and Wales whereas from the middle 1960s illegitimacy was notably higher in Dundee.

Only regional abortion rates are routinely available and Figure 2.2b shows that whereas Grampian (including Aberdeen) had the highest rate in the mid 1970s and has shown greater fluctuations, it has remained higher than that for Scotland; in the 1980s, however, it has been lower than that for Tayside (including Dundee) where in recent years the higher rate has been more comparable to that for England and Wales.

Figure 2.3 compares certain vital statistics for Aberdeen with the other three major cities in Scotland and nationally for the study years, 1951 and 1985. All cities and Scotland overall show marked falls in birth and stillbirth rates, but a considerable increase in illegitimacy. In both years, Aberdeen had an intermediate birth rate fairly similar to that for Edinburgh and lower than that for Scotland; the rate remained highest in Glasgow (Figure 2.3a). In 1951 the stillbirth rate was lowest in Aberdeen and highest in Glasgow, whereas in 1985 the two cities had similar high rates, above the rate for Scotland (Figure 2.3b). The proportion of Aberdeen births which were illegitimate was intermediate for the Scottish cities in both years, very similar to that for Edinburgh and slightly above the national percentage; the proportion remained highest in Dundee (Figure 2.3c).

It may be concluded that Aberdeen experience has been fairly typical of that elsewhere. Early notable differences, e.g. low stillbirth rate and high induced abortion rate have disappeared and in 1985 it is Dundee with its high rates of illegitimacy and induced abortion coupled with a low perinatal mortality which is more atypical.

2. The Sample

In order to assess the representativeness of the samples, primiparae for the years 1951 and 1985 will be considered, as these were the years in which most of the selected women were delivered.

TABLE 2.1

ALL ABERDEEN PRIMIPARAE, 1951 and 1985

	1951			1985		
	No.		%	No.		%
Single women	95		8.3	247		22.3
Married Previous pregnancy	72		6.3	197		17.7

First pregnancy
  Eligible for study
  Private patient
  Domiciliary patient
  Suburban resident
	824⎫
	66⎪
	24⎬ 973
	59⎭
			72.3⎫
			5.8⎪
			2.1⎬ 85.4
			5.2⎭
				658⎫
				7⎪
				—⎬ 665
				—⎭
						59.4⎫
						0.6⎪
						—⎬ 60.0
						—⎭

Total	1140		100.0	1109		100.0

Table 2.1 shows that nearly three times as many primiparae were single in 1985 as in 1951; also nearly three times as many married women had had a previous pregnancy the difference being almost entirely accounted for by induced abortions. Thus, whereas 85% of primiparae in 1951 were married and their first pregnancy had ended in a birth, this applied to only 60% in 1985. All these were not available for selection as private patients were excluded and in 1951 some women were delivered at home and others lived in the suburban areas which were later incorporated into the Aberdeen City District.

Thus, it is estimated that the samples studied came from 72% in 1951 and 59% in 1985 of all Aberdeen primiparae.

In considering how representative the samples were it is proposed to compare them with all married, primiparae (first pregnancy) i.e. with 973 women in 1951 and 665 women in 1985.

Only a proportion of the 1951 sample took part in the diet survey and in both studies the dietary data of a few women had to be discarded (see Chapter 11). It is, therefore, necessary to establish whether the women whose social and dietary data have been analysed were separately representative of married primiparae (first pregnancy).

Tables 2.2 and 2.3 summarise the findings in comparing the social and obstetric characteristics of the diet and social samples with each other and each with the married primiparae (first pregnancy) in the two years.

Table 2.2 shows that the 1951 diet and social samples were very similar to each other and to the total in all social and obstetric characteristics compared except that there were significantly fewer wives of non-manual workers in both samples. This is totally accounted for by the exclusion of private patients who were not eligible for selection.

TABLE 2.2

CHARACTERISTICS OF 1951 DIET AND SOCIAL SAMPLES AND 1951 TOTAL
MARRIED PRIMIPARAE (FIRST PREGNANCY)

		Diet (D)	Social (S)	Total (T)	Significant difference
(n)		94	213	973	
Social					
*	% brought up in Aberdeen	68.2	73.2	72.1	NS
†	% left school at minimum age	80.6	83.6	84.9	NS
*	% wife professional or clerical worker	33.2	29.6	30.2	NS
	% non-manual occupations				
*	wife's father	22.3	17.6	24.6	NS
*	husband	18.1	18.3	26.8	D v T p ⩽ 0.02
					S v T p ⩽ 0.02
†	% conceived prenuptially	31.4	26.3	26.4	NS
	Mean ages				
#	at marriage	22.8	22.4	22.6	NS
#	at delivery—wife	24.2	23.9	24.2	NS
#	—husband	26.5	26.6	26.4	NS
#	Mean maternal height (cm)	159.9	158.7	158.1	NS
Obstetric					
†	% labour not induced	86.1	84.0	88.7	NS
†	% spontaneous delivery	80.1	76.6	78.0	NS
†	% livebirths—singletons only	96.8	97.1	97.2	NS
#	Mean birthweight (g)	3204.6	3202.6	3205.9	NS
#	Mean gestation (completed weeks)	39.4	39.1	39.1	NS

Significance is based on:
* λ^2 distributions in accordance with detailed analysis in following chapters
† λ^2 dichotomous classification
# t test

Table 2.3 shows that the 1985 diet and social samples are representative of the total in most social and all obstetric characteristics. However, the diet sample had a slight excess of women who were professional and clerical workers and a deficit of husbands in non-manual occupations; in contrast the social sample had a slight excess of non-manual worker husbands and a deficit of women in professional and clerical occupations. Further investigation indicates that these differences may be artifacts. In 1951 the occupational data for the samples and total were obtained by the research team whereas in 1985 data for the total were recorded by specially trained clerical staff at routine clinic interviews and details of education and training

TABLE 2.3

CHARACTERISTICS OF 1985 DIET AND SOCIAL SAMPLES AND 1985 TOTAL MARRIED PRIMIPARAE (FIRST PREGNANCY)

		Diet (D)	Social (S)	Total (T)	Significant difference
(n)		142	158	665	
Social					
*	% brought up in Aberdeen	57.0	57.0	55.9	NS
†	% left school at minimum age	42.3	43.7	47.4	NS
*	% wife professional or clerical worker	73.6	71.5	73.0	S v T p ≤ 0.02 D v T p ≤ 0.05
	% non-manual occupations				
*	wife's father	42.1	43.1	32.5	NS
*	husband	40.8	43.0	41.7	S v T p ≤ 0.05 D v T p ≤ 0.02
†	% conceived prenuptially	9.0	6.3	15.1	S v T p ≤ 0.02
	Mean ages				
#	at marriage	22.7	22.7	21.6	NS
#	at delivery—wife	25.6	25.5	25.1	NS
#	—husband	28.0	27.9	25.9	NS
#	Mean maternal height (cm)	161.6	161.1	161.1	NS
Obstetric					
†	% labour not induced	61.2	60.1	64.5	NS
†	% spontaneous delivery	52.1	51.9	54.4	NS
†	% livebirth—singletons only	96.5	98.1	99.2	NS
#	Mean birthweight (g)	3232.6	3185.6	3232.4	NS
#	Mean gestation (completed weeks)	39.3	39.2	39.3	NS

Significance is based on:
* λ^2 distributions in accordance with detailed analysis in following chapters
† λ^2 dichotomous classification
# t test

were not always available to allow precise classification comparable to the research data.

In general, therefore, the samples can be taken as representative of married primiparae (first pregnancy) in the early 1950s and mid 1980s. The significance of illegitimacy and abortion in starting a family in the intervening decades has been reported elsewhere (Pritchard and Thompson, 1982: Thompson *et al.*, 1984).

FIGURE 2.1 a, b, c RATES 1950–85 IN 3 YEAR AVERAGES FOR
ABERDEEN, DUNDEE, SCOTLAND AND ENGLAND AND WALES

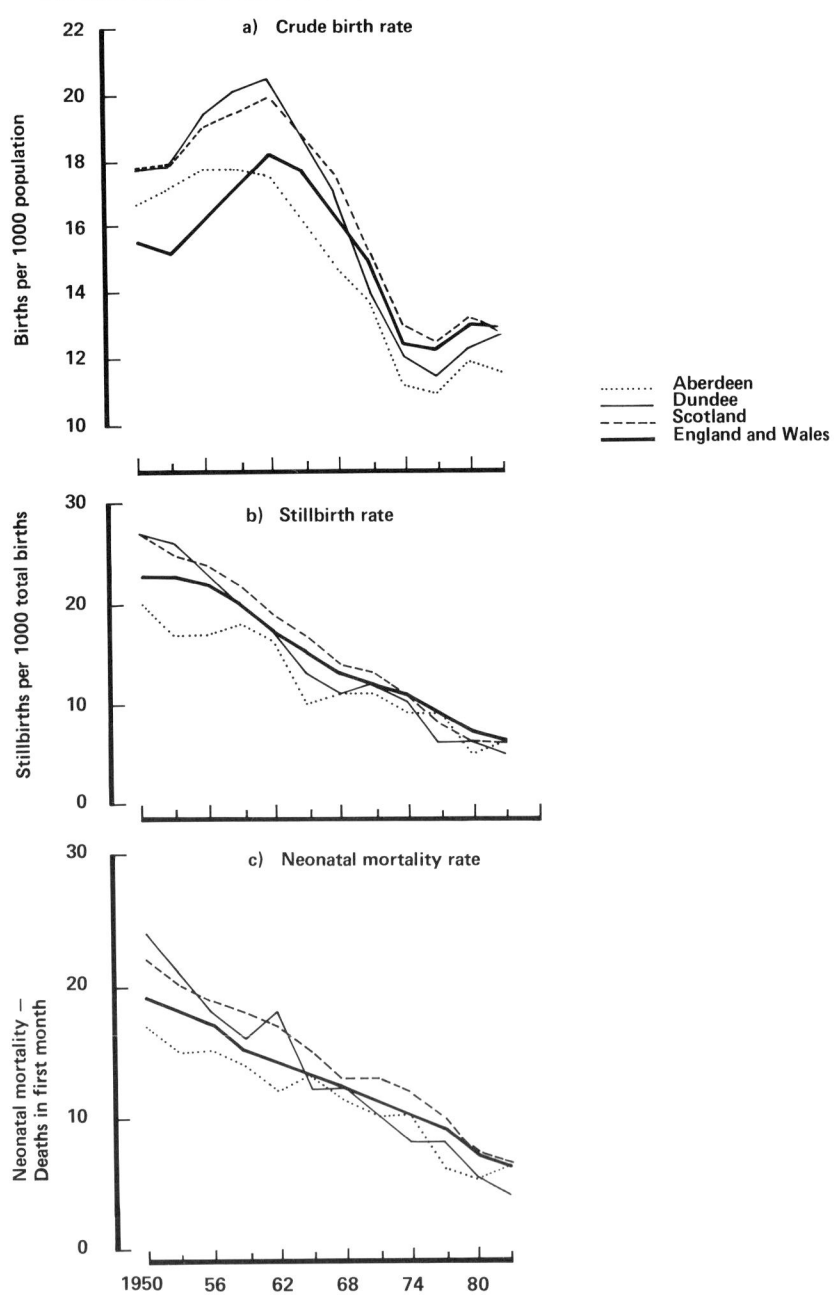

FIGURE 2.2 a, b FACTORS AFFECTING WOMEN AVAILABLE FOR SELECTION IN ABERDEEN STUDIES

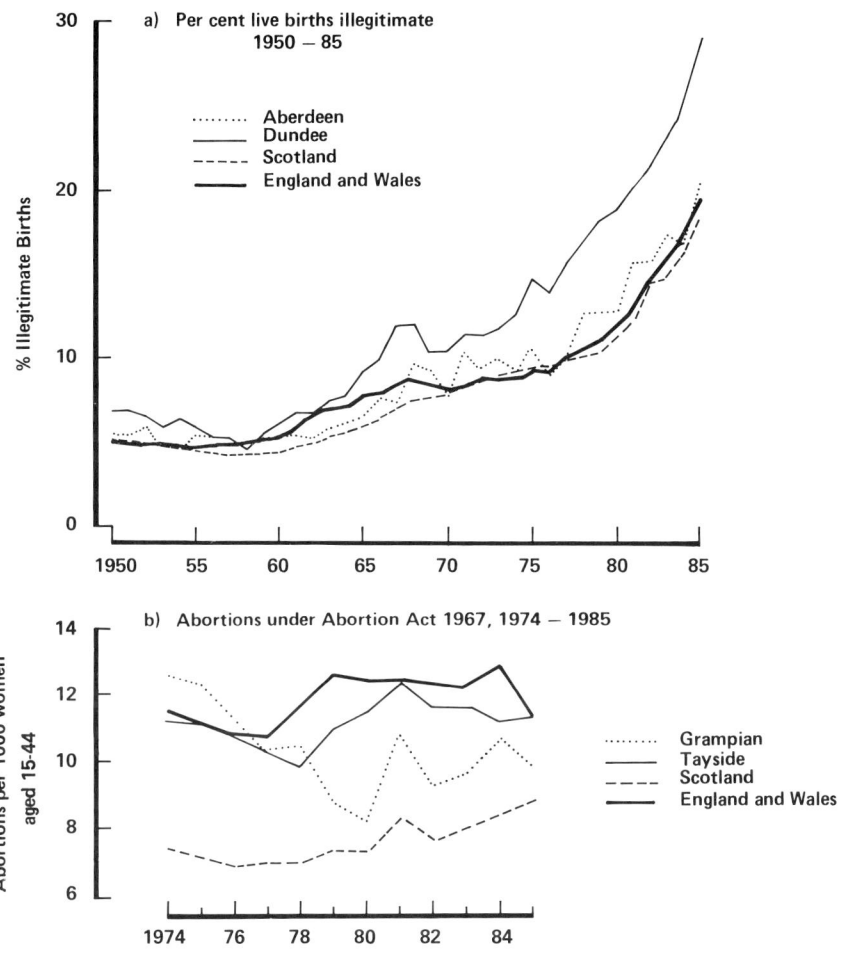

a) Per cent live births illegitimate 1950 – 85

.... Aberdeen
——— Dundee
– – – – Scotland
━━━━ England and Wales

b) Abortions under Abortion Act 1967, 1974 – 1985

.... Grampian
——— Tayside
– – – – Scotland
━━━━ England and Wales

(*see facing page*)

The Sources for Figures 2.1 a, b, and c were:

Registrar General Scotland, Annual Reports 1950–85 (Edinburgh HMSO) Scottish Health Service, Scottish Health Statistics, Annual Reports 1974–85 (Edinburgh, HMSO)

Registrar General's Statistical Review of England and Wales, Annual Reports 1950–73 (London, HMSO)

Office of Population Censuses and Surveys, Birth Statistics for England and Wales, Annual Reports 1974–85 (London, HMSO)

Office of Population Censuses and Surveys, Abortion Statistics for England and Wales, Annual Reports 1974–85 (London, HMSO)

FIGURE 2.3 a, b, c   BIRTH STATISTICS FOR ABERDEEN COMPARED WITH OTHER SCOTTISH CITIES AND SCOTLAND FOR 1951 AND 1985

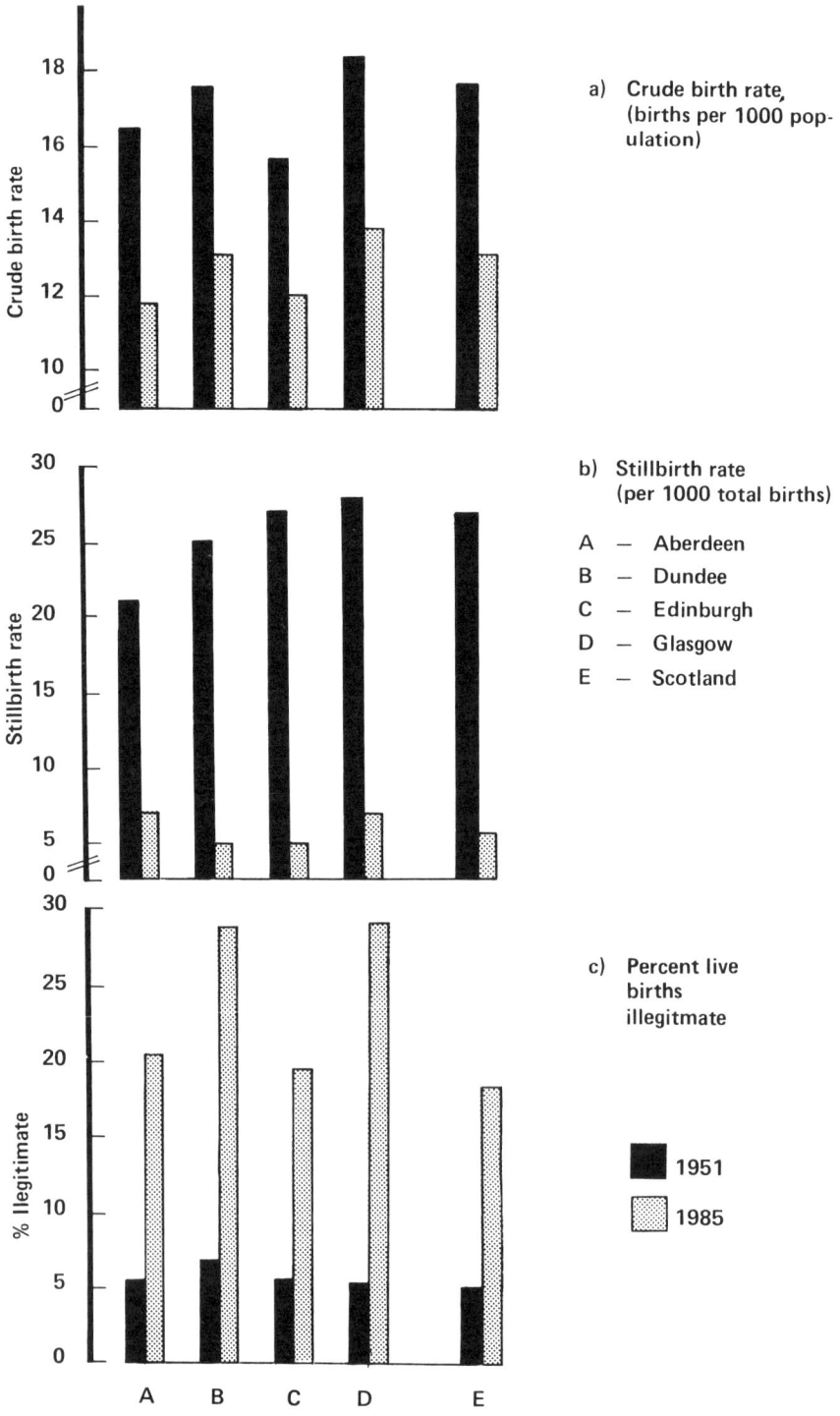

a) Crude birth rate, (births per 1000 population)

b) Stillbirth rate (per 1000 total births)

A — Aberdeen
B — Dundee
C — Edinburgh
D — Glasgow
E — Scotland

c) Percent live births illegitmate

■ 1951

▨ 1985

## CHAPTER 3

Social Background of the Couples

The 1951 and 1985 samples of married primigravidae were significantly different in respect of the limited social factors considered in Chapter 2. In this chapter some aspects of the social background of the couples will be considered in more detail and compared for the two samples.

Place of Origin or Upbringing

The 1951 sample of primigravidae was predominantly of local origin with 70% of both wives and husbands having been born in Aberdeen, where the vast majority had also been brought up (Table 3.1). Although over half the couples in the 1985 sample had also been born and bred in Aberdeen, the greater diversity in their places of origin and upbringing is statistically significant compared with the earlier sample, especially in respect of the wives. A detailed study of the motivation and characteristics of migrants amongst all Aberdeen married primigravidae 1952–9 has been published elsewhere (Illsley *et al.*, 1963*a*).

TABLE 3.1

PLACE OF BIRTH AND UPBRINGING

Birth	Brought up	Wife		Husband	
		1951	1985	1951	1985
(n)		(213)	(158)	(131)*	(158)
		%	%	%	%
Aberdeen	Aberdeen	69	55	68	52
Aberdeen	Other	1	2	2	4
Other	Aberdeen	8	6	5	8
Other	Grampian	12	9	12	7
Other	Rest Scotland	5	18	9	17
Other	Elsewhere	5	10	4	12
Total		100	100	100	100

$$\lambda_{(5)}^2 = 22.62 \quad p \leqslant 0.001 \qquad \lambda_{(5)}^2 = 16.48 \quad p \leqslant 0.01$$

* excludes 82 as initially husband's place of birth not recorded

Most of the women and their husbands born outside Aberdeen were brought up in the area where they were born. Table 3.1 shows that over the 34 year period there had been a decrease in immigrants to Aberdeen from the Grampian Region and a substantial increase in those coming from the rest of Scotland or from 'elsewhere'. Detailed examination of the records show that whereas in 1951 'elsewhere' referred almost exclusively to England, in 1985 nearly half those who came from 'elsewhere' were from abroad. This applied to only one wife (from Argentina) and no husbands in the 1951 sample, whereas in the 1985 sample, ten wives and eight husbands came from overseas. Eight of the ten wives were foreign nationals from Australia (2), India, Iraq, Japan, the Netherlands, Pakistan and Trinidad; the remaining two were British nationals born in Malaysia and Pakistan who had returned to England for their secondary education. Of the eight husbands three, like their wives included above, were foreign nationals from Australia, Iraq and the Netherlands; the remaining five were all British nationals who had come to Britain from Hong Kong (2); South Africa; West Germany; and Zambia.

These significant changes in places of birth and upbringing reflect the emergence of Aberdeen as a major centre in the world's oil industry; many multinational oil and related service companies have set up offices in Aberdeen and have brought key workers to the area.

Family of Upbringing

The details of upbringing were important in pinpointing the chief wage earner in the family and, therefore, in determining the socio-economic conditions or social class of upbringing. The significance of a broken home and of different types of upbringing to women in Aberdeen has been reported in detail elsewhere (Illsley and Thompson, 1961; Edwards and Thompson, 1971).

It should be remembered that the couples in the 1951 sample had lived through the 1939–45 War and some of their families had suffered. For example, the father of four primigravidae had been killed and a further six fathers had become war pensioners, with limited opportunity for employment due to disabilities such as blindness or loss of a limb.

TYPE OF UPBRINGING

The women and their husbands were considered to have had a 'usual' upbringing if they had lived with both their natural parents up to school leaving age. This applied to significantly more primigravidae in 1985 than in 1951 (Table 3.2), but the principal reason for 'other' family situations had changed between the studies—the death of a parent predominated in the earlier study, whereas separation and divorce of parents was the main reason in 1985. The pattern for husbands was similar, but the difference was not significant. It may be noted, however, that a few women could not be precise

TABLE 3.2

TYPE OF UPBRINGING

Type	Wife		Husband	
	1951	1985	1951	1985
(n)	(213)	(158)	(208)*	(157)*
	%	%	%	%
Usual	80	89	83	86
Other				
Parent(s) died	12	3	13	6
Father	7.5⎫	2.5⎫	7⎫	5⎫
Mother	4 ⎬	0.5⎭	5 ⎬	1⎭
Both	0.5⎭		1 ⎭	
Parents separated or divorced	1	4	1	6
Fostered/adopted	3	1	1	1
Miscellaneous	4	3	2	1
Total	100	100	100	100
Usual v other	$\lambda^2_{(1)} = 5.76$	$p \leqslant 0.02$	$\lambda^2_{(1)} = 1.47$	NS

* Excluding not stated

about their husband's upbringing, especially if they had not known him for very long or had not met his family.

The pattern of parental death is what might be expected from the differential mortality of men and women and the increased expectation of life over time. In both studies more fathers than mothers had died. None of the 1985 primigravidae or their husbands had lost both parents. Arrangements made after the death of a parent were very similar in the two periods. When the father died, the child had usually stayed with the mother, a minority of whom remarried. Death of a mother had been more disruptive of family life and to some extent the women and their husbands had been differently affected. Although most had remained with their fathers, much depended on the age at which they had lost their mother, and also the availability of a female relative, e.g. older sister or grandmother. None of the women had been sent to an institution after their mother died, whereas this, and also boarding out, had happened to husbands in both samples. Sometimes living arrangements had changed when the father remarried.

The few women or husbands in the 1951 sample whose parents had been divorced or separated had all stayed with their mother; the fathers had gone away. This did not always apply in the 1985 sample, and some mothers had left home. A few children had remained throughout with their father and others had rejoined him either when he remarried or circumstances changed, e.g. mother became ill or died. Grandparents often helped out and there had been occasional temporary fostering.

Illegitimacy was nearly always the reason for permanent fostering or adoption. Illegitimate children kept by their mother had usually been incorporated into her parental home, and had often stayed there after she had married. 'Other' types of upbringing also includes those where the parents lived abroad—in 1951 this only applied to husbands left behind when their parents emigrated, whereas in 1985 both wives and husbands had been sent to school in Britain. Wartime evacuation had only affected one 1951 primigravida who only returned home when she left school.

CHIEF WAGE EARNER

The father was classified as the chief wage earner in the case of 'usual' upbringing and in some of the 'other' types, depending on the age in childhood when any disruption of the family had occurred and the circumstances. For example, if the father died when the child was aged three and the mother went out to work thereafter, she would be coded as the chief wage earner, whereas the father would be taken as the chief wage earner if he had not died until the child was aged 13; if an illegitimate child became part of the mother's parental family, then the grandfather might be coded as the chief wage earner. Obviously, in a few cases an arbitrary decision had to be taken about the relevant classification particularly where there had been several changes in the living arrangements, e.g. if a father deserted the family and the child went to live with grandparents, but later rejoined the mother and a step-father.

In most cases the father was identified as the chief wage earner—in 89% and 94% of the families of the primigravidae in the 1951 and 1985 samples

TABLE 3.3

OCCUPATION OF CHIEF WAGE EARNER

Occupation	Wife		Husband	
(n)	1951 (210)* %	1985 (158) %	1951 (202)* %	1985 (151)* %
Male				
non-manual	18	42	21	31
skilled manual	36	31	41	41
other manual	41	24	35	24
Female	5	3	3	4
Total	100	100	100	100
	$\lambda^2_{(3)} = 28.04$ $p \leqslant 0.001$		$\lambda^2_{(3)} = 6.70$ Not significant	

* Excluding not stated

respectively. Comparable figures for the husbands were 93% and 94% respectively. Half the remaining chief wage earners were other males; in 1951 it was usually a grandfather whereas in 1985 it was more likely to be a step-father. Other male chief wage earners included uncles, foster and adoptive fathers. Females, normally mothers, were the chief wage earner in the remainder of families. No classification could be made for a few confused or institutional upbringings or when data were incomplete.

Table 3.3 shows that significantly more wives in the 1985 sample had been brought up in households headed by a non-manual worker. Fewer came from homes where the chief wage earner was in a semi-skilled or unskilled manual job or was a woman. For the husbands the trend was similar, but not significant.

FAMILY SIZE

Both the primigravidae and their husbands in the recent sample came from significantly smaller families than those in the 1951 sample (Table 3.4). More of the men and women in 1985 than in 1951 had one or two brothers and sisters. The proportion of only children remained fairly constant.

MATERNAL HEIGHT

Height may be taken as an indication of the social and environmental circumstances in which a child has been raised. The stunted, rachitic children found in overcrowded city slums earlier this century are a notorious

TABLE 3.4

SIZE OF FAMILY OF UPBRINGING

No. of children (n)	Wife		Husband	
	1951 (213) %	1985 (158) %	1951 (206)* %	1985 (158) %
1	5	5	9	6
2	18	26	15	25
3	16	31	21	30
4 or over	57	37	53	39
Variable/Institution	4	1	2	—
Total	100	100	100	100
Mean	4.30 ± 2.06	3.23 ± 1.36	4.21 ± 2.18	3.32 ± 1.47
	$t = 5.65$	$p \leqslant 0.001$	$t = 4.40$	$p \leqslant 0.001$

* Excluding not stated

TABLE 3.5

MATERNAL HEIGHT

(n)	1951 (213) %	1985 (158) %
Short—under 1.55m	22	13
Medium—1.55 to 1.62m	55	43
Tall—1.63m and over	23	44
Total	100	100

$$\lambda^2_{(2)} = 18.73 \quad p \leqslant 0.001$$

Mean height m	1.587 ± 0.066	1.616 ± 0.063

$$t = 4.13 \quad p \leqslant 0.001$$

example. Although genetic factors are important in physical development and adult height, achieving growth potential depends on many factors, including nutrition and health (Hytten and Leitch, 1971). In the early 1950s many studies from Aberdeen (e.g. Baird, 1952; Baird and Illsley, 1953) showed that maternal height increased with socio-economic status and the phenomenon is now generally established. Any deprivation which might lead to stunting in growth and adversely affect the shape of the pelvis has important obstetric implication In studying this problem, Bernard (1952) divided Aberdeen women into three height groups—short, medium and tall, the cut-off points being under 5'1" and 5'4" and over, giving approximately 25, 50 and 25 per cent respectively.

Using this same broad classification, Table 3.5 shows that there has been a significant change in the height of married primigravidae over the years— the proportion of tall women (1.63m and over) almost doubled while that of short women (under 1.55m) fell by about one third. This change is reflected in the highly significant increase in mean height by nearly three centimetres. But this is not merely a feature of these selected married primigravidae, but applies to all Aberdeen women having a first baby (Fraser, 1987)

Education

Between the two studies there had been a highly significant change in the educational experience of both the primigravidae and their husbands (Table 3.6). Compared with 1951, only about half as many in the 1985 sample had left school at the minimum age, notwithstanding that this had been raised from 15 to 16 in the intervening years. Most wives and husbands in the recent sample had stayed on at school or gone on to further technical, professional or academic training. One in five of the primigravidae had been

TABLE 3.6

EDUCATION

	Wife		Husband	
	1951	1985	1951	1985
(n)	(213)	(158)	(209)*	(158)
	%	%	%	%
Left school				
Minimum age	84	44	88	48
Later	9	16	6	18
Further training				
Technical	5	20	2	11
University	2	20	4	23
Total	100	100	100	100

$\lambda^2_{(3)} = 73.50 \quad p \leqslant 0.001$ $\lambda^2_{(3)} = 70.77 \quad p \leqslant 0.001$

* Excluding not stated

to University or its equivalent, a ten fold increase compared with the earlier sample.

The Married Couple

The age at which the 1985 sample of primigravidae had married was significantly concentrated in the early 20s, nearly two-thirds compared with less than half in the earlier sample; fewer had married in their teens or after

TABLE 3.7

AGE AT MARRIAGE—WIFE AND HUSBAND

Age at marriage	Wife		Husband	
(Years)	1951	1985	1951	1985
(n)	(213)	(158)	(213)	(158)
	%	%	%	%
-19	28	13	3	3
20-24	48	61	54	56
25-29	17	22	31	28
30 and over	7	4	12	13
Total	100	100	100	100

$\lambda^2_{(3)} = 14.04 \quad p \leqslant 0.001$ $\lambda^2_{(3)} = 0.47 \text{ Not significant}$

age 30 (Table 3.7). The mean ages, however, were very similar—22.4 in 1951 and 22.6 in 1985.

The age of husbands at marriage showed no significant change, over half in each sample being in their early 20s and about one in eight being over age 30 (Table 3.7). The husbands remained on average two to two-and-a-half years older than the wives. The ways in which the couples had originally met had not changed significantly (Table 3.8). A casual meeting was the most usual way in both studies, often at the dance hall (1951) or disco (1985). Over one-fifth of the couples in each sample had met at work or at college or University. A few couples in the 1951 sample had met while both were serving in the Forces.

Some couples had known each other all their lives, while others were married soon after they had met. A fairly similar proportion, about one-seventh, in each sample had married within one year. On average, couples in both samples had known each other about three-and-a half years before marrying, and the difference was not significant.

A feature in the 1985 study, however, was that 22% of the primigravidae

TABLE 3.8

HOW WIFE MET HUSBAND

How met	1951	1985
(n)	(103)*	(158)
	%	%
Known as children		
Same school	4	8
Families friends/		
neighbours	14	1
Later		
Youth/Recreation Club	8	3
As adult		
Work/University etc	23	22
Introduced by friends/		
relatives	15	23
Casual		
Dancing/disco	18	28
Other	13	10
Miscellaneous	5	5
Total	100	100

$$\lambda^2_{(5)} = 9.52 \text{ Not significant}$$

* Excluding initial 110 for whom no information

reported having lived with their husbands for periods of up to seven years before they married, and this is likely to be a minimum as there was considerable evidence to suggest that others may also have cohabited. Of those who reported cohabitation two-thirds said they had lived together for less than a year and nearly one quarter for three or more years. This meant that of the total sample, 14% reported that they had cohabited for up to a year, 3% for one to three years, and 5% for three or more years before they married. The question was not even considered in the 1950s, and the housing situation in Aberdeen would have militated against it (see Chapter 4). There had been some long engagements in the earlier sample, as couples waited to marry until they obtained a home of their own. By contrast some young men and women in the recent sample had lived independently in property they owned or rented.

Marriage during pregnancy showed a significant decline undoubtedly due to the revolution in the use of contraception over the years (see Chapter 6). Whereas 26% of women in the 1951 sample had had a prenuptial conception (PNC) this applied to 6% in the recent sample. Also 'honeymoon' pregnancies had halved (Table 3.9). In contrast, compared with the 1951 sample, twice as many couples in 1985 had been married at least a year before pregnancy occurred so that this now applied to the majority.

TABLE 3.9

INTERVAL BETWEEN MARRIAGE AND LAST MENSTRUAL PERIOD

(n)	1951 (213) %	1985 (158) %
LMP 4 weeks or more before marriage (prenuptial conception)	26	6
LMP 3 weeks before to 3 weeks after marriage ('honeymoon' conception)	11	5
LMP after marriage completed months		
1-2	14	10
3-5	14	10
6-11	11	16
12 and over	24	53
Total	100	100

$$\lambda^2_{(5)} = 50.42 \quad p \leqslant 0.001$$

CHAPTER 4

Housing

All the primigravidae in the 1951 sample lived within the City of Aberdeen, whereas only 98 of the 158 primigravidae in the recent study lived in the same area. The remaining 60 women resided in the suburban areas now included in the geographically defined Aberdeen City District as described in Chapter 1.

Details of their housing conditions and living arrangements were discussed with the women at the ANC, supplemented in the earlier study by a home visit. Six items were considered:

1. Ownership
2. Tenancy
3. Type of house
4. Sanitary facilities
5. Domestic living and cooking arrangements
6. Persons per room

Analysis of the data shows that in the years between the two studies, significant changes had occurred in all aspects of the housing of these married couples expecting their first baby. Table 4.1 shows that in the 1985 sample the majority of couples owned their own home (72%). This was exceptional in the 1951 sample (4%) when typically the couples lived in sublet accommodation (62%) almost half of them in one room in the wife's parental home.

In the early 1950s there was an acute housing shortage in Aberdeen and few young couples were in a position to buy property which came on the market. The Town Council was engaged in slum clearance projects, and was rapidly developing housing estates on the outskirts of the city, but these council houses were allocated on points given for family size and composition, lack of facilities and medical requirements. The situation was so severe that couples usually had to have two children before they were likely to qualify (Thompson, 1954). Although 87 of the 213 primigravidae in the earlier study lived in council property, only 3 were tenants, the rest subletting from tenants usually their parents or in-laws. In contrast, in the recent sample, 23 of the 158 couples lived in council property and 17 of them were tenants.

The majority of the 1951 couples lived in privately owned property, but only 32% were tenants, the remaining 23% being in sublet rooms. The

28

TABLE 4.1

HOUSING—OWNERSHIP AND TENANCY

(n)		1951 (213) %	1985 (158) %
Ownership			
Owner and occupier		4	72
Private		55	10
Council		40.5	14
Tied		0.5	4
		$\lambda^2_{(3)} = 204.65$ p $\leqslant 0.001$	
Tenancy			
Owned		4	72
Rented unfurnished		29	16
Sublet from—			
wife's parents	29 ⎫		4 ⎫
husband's parents	10 ⎬ 62		1 ⎬ 8
other relatives	9 ⎪		3 ⎪
strangers	14 ⎭		— ⎭
Other		5	4
Total		100	100
		$\lambda^2_{(3)} = 201.32$ p $\leqslant 0.001$	

chances of renting private property were facilitated if someone could 'speak for them', e.g. if parents had a private landlord who could be persuaded to give a forthcoming vacant tenancy to a son or daughter. Many women 'did the rounds' of housing factors in an attempt to get their name on waiting lists, or followed up any property likely to become vacant as a result of death or a removal. Some soon gave up this soul destroying effort and decided to wait for a council house. In contrast, in 1985, only one tenth of the couples lived in privately owned property, 6% were tenants and 4% lived in sublet rooms.

Houses tied to the husband's work had increased from 0.5% in the earlier study to 4% in 1985. The University featured at both times, but more recently the police, the army, oil companies and a religious organisation were involved.

As so many primigravidae in the 1985 sample were owner occupiers or tenants in unfurnished property (88% compared with 33% in 1951), so the proportion who lived in sublet rooms had fallen (from 62% in 1951 to 8%). Typically in 1951 the couples lived with the wife's parents, or less frequently with her in-laws, or with other relatives, e.g. sisters, aunts. Nearly one-seventh, however, shared with strangers, i.e. unrelated persons; but none lived in these conditions in 1985.

In the recent study, of the 12 couples who were in sublet rooms, seven were in the wife's parental home, one was with the husband's parents and the remaining four were with other relatives. With the exception of one couple who lived with the wife's widowed father, they were all on the council waiting list, and one couple had felt confident enough to turn down the offer of a flat, preferring to wait for a house which they expected to get before the baby was born.

A small proportion of couples in each sample had 'other' tenancy arrangements which included furnished accommodation and covered some of the 'tied' houses in the recent sample. One couple in the earlier study, because of exceptional circumstances, had a joint tenancy of a council house with the wife's parents.

Although in both studies the majority of the couples lived in flats, there had been a significant fall (82% to 53%) in favour of self-contained houses, and in particular the proportion of semi-detached houses had almost trebled (Table 4.2). In the 1985 sample one couple lived in a residential caravan.

Many of the flats in 1951 were in traditional Scottish tenements with shared wc on the stairway or outside the building. Only 53% of couples in

TABLE 4.2

HOUSING TYPE AND FACILITIES

(n)	1951 (213) %	1985 (158) %
Type		
Detached	3	6
Semi-detached	11	29
Terraced	4	11
Flat, tenement	82	53
Other	—	1
Total	100	100

$$\lambda^2_{(4)} = 34.57 \quad p \leqslant 0.001$$

	1951	1985
Facilities		
Modern conveniences	53	98
wc on stair	22	2
wc outside	25	—
Total	100	100

$$\lambda^2_{(2)} = 92.17 \quad p \leqslant 0.001$$

the earlier sample lived in a home with modern conveniences, i.e. running hot and cold water, bath and wc, which was typically a shared council house. In the 1985 sample, only three couples lacked modern conveniences and all expected to be rehoused by the Council by the time the baby arrived—two were already council tenants, but the third was living in the most insanitary conditions in private property.

With the prevalence of sublet accommodation in the 1951 sample more overcrowding would be anticipated. Indeed, the average number of persons per room in 1951 was 1.35 compared with only 0.73 in 1985, a highly significant statistical difference ($p \leqslant 0.001$).

Typically in the early 1950s the couple had to rely on their parents, usually the wife's, to give them a room. If they had to go elsewhere they would often return when a married sibling with children moved out on being allocated a council house. In one case, the pressures on the parental homes were so great that the couple, married during pregnancy, had never lived together, but remained with their respective parents. The parental home was the refuge to which couples turned in a crisis, e.g. a couple turned out of their sublet with strangers when the landlady found out about the pregnancy, went to the wife's home. This meant that her parents and two brothers had to sleep in the living room which led to rows. The data analysed refer to the houses where the couple slept, but in seven cases the couple virtually lived elsewhere, spending the day, having all meals, doing their washing, etc., in the mother or mother-in-law's already crowded house. This was necessary because of the inadequate facilities or difficulties with landladies in sublets from strangers. As indicated above some women had to face the threat of eviction when their pregnancy became obvious or were told that they could not return to their accommodation with the baby. Given the unpredictable situations, the poor facilities and overcrowding in which many primigravidae lived, it is not surprising that housing was their main concern in the early 1950s.

Most couples in the recent sample lived on their own and were independent in their living arrangements (Table 4.3), having sole responsibility for domestic chores and cooking (90%). Those in sublet accommodation tended to be semi-dependent, i.e. doing their own cooking but sharing household facilities. The arrangements for five couples, however, were classed as anomalous—two had bought large houses and were running them as boarding houses, one wife acted as housekeeper for her widowed father, and the living arrangements of the other two couples varied as a result of men working offshore; one woman always went to stay with her mother when her husband was offshore, and one couple had the house to themselves when their unmarried landlord was offshore.

In the 1951 sample the living arrangements were significantly different as just over one-third lived independently and nearly one-fifth had no domestic responsibilities as they boarded with the family with whom they lived. Nearly one-third maintained some independence in a shared home, whereas one in seven lived in 'anomalous' circumstances. These latter included those couples who lived and slept in different houses, or whose conditions

TABLE 4.3

LIVING ARRANGEMENTS

	1951	1985
(n)	(213)	(158)
	%	%
Living arrangements		
Independent	36	90
Semi-dependent	31	7
Boarding	19	—
Anomalous	14	3
Total	100	100

$$\lambda^2_{(3)} = 110.71 \quad p \leqslant 0.001$$

fluctuated, but the majority had additional housekeeping responsibilities for the person or family with whom they shared including catering for a widowed father or father-in-law, an aged mother or handicapped landlady or female relatives who worked full-time.

The increased mobility of the 1985 couples as well as the availability of housing is reflected in the number of homes they had had. Table 4.4 shows that significantly more couples in the 1985 sample had lived together in more than one home—on average 1.85 homes, compared with 1.38 in the earlier sample. More than twice as many couples in the recent sample had lived in three or more homes.

Typically in the recent survey the couples had started out buying a small flat, or one or other partner had already owned a home and the other had moved in. Moves were usually to a larger property, the preferred choices

TABLE 4.4

NUMBER OF HOMES

	1951	1985
(n)	(204)*	(158)
	%	%
Homes		
0	0.5	—
1	70	42
2	23	43
3+	6.5	15
Total	100	100

$$\lambda^2_{(2)} = 29.34 \quad p \leqslant 0.001$$

* Data incomplete for 9 couples

being a semi-detached, terraced or detached house. A few couples who started out in rented accommodation had bought their own homes and some who were initially in sublet rooms had become council tenants. However, ten couples had lived in at least four homes, usually in a succession of tied or rented private accommodation—these included a soldier and his wife and two couples from overseas where the husbands' jobs in oil had meant a good deal of worldwide mobility. In contrast, the 1951 couples had usually started their life in sublet accommodation (usually in council property with modern conveniences, but in very overcrowded conditions—1.71 persons per room); or had found a home of their own in privately owned but sub-standard property (1.08 persons per room). Moves had seldom improved the couple's living conditions.

Housing conditions in the City of Aberdeen in the early 1950s were appalling. The new Medical Officer of Health (Dr I A G McQueen) in his annual report for 1952 stated ' . . . that it has a good deal of overcrowding; and that it compares unfavourably with the other principal cities of Scotland in the proportion of householders lacking piped water supplies, water closets, kitchen sinks and cooking facilities'. The 1951 Census had revealed the shattering finding that in some respects, Aberdeen was worse than Glasgow, which was notorious for its bad housing. The situation by the mid 1980s had been revolutionised. Some account of housing developments over the years and latterly of the impact of the oil industry has been given elsewhere (Payne, 1975). In the 1970s and early 1980s private housing developments mushroomed in the suburban areas providing a wide range of properties some of which specifically catered for young couples able to obtain a mortgage. Thus, for the married couples starting a family who participated in the recent study, independence in homes, well equipped to a high standard was the norm. It should be remembered, however, that these represented only 59% of all Aberdeen primigravidae and no information on the housing conditions of the remainder is available.

## CHAPTER 5

Contraception and Family Intentions

In the early 1950s contraception was an embarrassing subject even for professionals, and doctors seldom volunteered information. Any discussion was perfunctory and likely to be limited by nervous laughter. There was little publicity and many women were ill-informed about the different methods. The provision in Aberdeen was better than in most places elsewhere, as a voluntary organisation had provided contraception services since the 1930s (Baird, 1965). Enlightened, upper social class women, inspired by Marie Stopes, had established a clinic in a central, poor area of the city. However, most women remained unaware of the clinic, reflecting the general secrecy and ambiguity surrounding contraception.

In these early years, the methods available to couples were coitus interruptus, the sheath, safe period, chemicals and diaphragm. It was not until May 1964 that oral contraception was introduced into Aberdeen and the intra-uterine device (IUCD) followed soon after (Thompson, 1977).

When the 1951 study was carried out, the diaphragm was recommended as the safest method of contraception. It was fitted, other than in exceptional circumstances, at the Family Planning Clinic, euphemistically called the Gynaecological Advisory Clinic, which had been set up in the basement of the Antenatal Clinic when, in 1948, the Local Health Authority took over the services provided by the voluntary organisation. However, most women found the very idea of the diaphragm abhorrent and it was used by only a few primigravidae usually in the upper social classes (Illsley, 1956a; Thompson and Aitken-Swan, 1973; Thompson, 1977). At that time a small charge was made. There was no general publicity about the clinic and the psychologist found that many primigravidae had never heard of it or were misinformed. For example, some thought that only married women with at least two children could attend. The Local Health Authority abolished charges at the renamed Family Planning Clinic in 1966 before family planning became an integral part of the National Health Service (NHS).

By the time of the 1985 study contraception was available free under the National Health Service from the Family Planning Clinic or from general practitioners who received allowances for attending training courses and remuneration for providing contraceptive services. In addition, there had been extensive sex education programmes, and media publicity of all kinds on marriage and family planning. Aberdeen had pioneered television programmes on sex education for use in schools, which initially were presented by an obstetrician, but did not include the subject of contraception (Gill *et al.*, 1971).

Details of the contraceptive methods used by the couples were noted at the antenatal interviews. In the 1951 study this information was only available for 159 primigravidae who saw the psychologist, but data were complete for the 158 women in the 1985 study. Table 5.1 shows the dramatic change in use of contraception with the introduction of new methods between the surveys. Nearly all couples in the 1985 study had used contraception (95%) compared with less than half (43%) in 1951. Only eight of the 158 women in the recent sample said that they and their husbands had never used any form of contraception. These included four women, married up to 12 years, who wanted children and did not mind when they started a family, one who ovulated very infrequently and knew it would be difficult for her to become pregnant and three who had conceived prenuptially.

The majority of the earlier sample had never used contraception. Some of the women displayed considerable ignorance about methods available and talked of 'being green' or 'not knowing anything about that'. There were many misconceptions, such as the idea that pregnancy could not occur at first intercourse or if the woman did not enjoy coitus. Holding such beliefs a few women were 'shocked to have been caught'. Again, there was a great deal of fatalism, variously expressed in comments such as:

'If they are there you are meant to have them—I don't believe in birth control.'
'The first child shouldn't be prevented.'
'If it happens, it happens.'
'What will be, will be—if they do come in steps and stairs that's meant.'

TABLE 5.1

CONTRACEPTION EVER USED

(n)	1951 (159)*	1985 (158)
Method	% used method	% used method
None	57	5
Coitus interruptus	25	—
Sheath	13	29
Safe period	4	3
Chemicals alone	8	1
Diaphragm	2	4
IUCD	Not available	4
Pill	Not available	91

* Excludes 54 women not seen by psychologist

Such sentiments were never expressed by women in the 1985 sample. In marked contrast these primigravidae accepted that a couple could control fairly precisely the timing and spacing of children, barring medical problems, and some of them had already decided on which partner would be sterilised when their families were complete.

In the 1950s the most popular contraceptive method was coitus interruptus which had been tried by about one quarter of couples whereas it was not reported as used by any couples in the 1985 sample. By this time the pill had revolutionised contraceptive practice and it had been used by 91% of the primigravidae who took part in the recent study. In fact, of the 150 couples who had used contraception only six wives had never taken the pill, preferring 'not to play around with hormones', but to rely on mechanical methods. The sheath was the second most popular method in both samples, but the proportion of couples who had used it had more than doubled (13% in 1951; 29% in 1985). Various types of chemical preparations on their own, in the form of foams and creams had reportedly been used by 8% of the 1951 sample, but by none in the 1985 sample, although one woman had used pessaries. No couple in either sample had relied entirely on the safe period although a few had used it for varying lengths of time usually in conjunction with other methods. In the earlier study some of the women had not fully understood instructions and had had intercourse at their most fertile time, but there was no evidence of this in the recent study. The unpopular diaphragm had been used by only 2% of women in 1951, and by 4% of the 1985 sample. A similar proportion of women in 1985 had had an IUCD fitted.

Given the very limited choice available in the 1950s, the great majority of those who had used contraception had tried only one method. No couples in either study reported using more than three methods, but the greater experience of the 1985 sample is evident in that 33% said they had tried two or three methods compared with 7% in the earlier sample.

FIRST CHOICE AND SEQUENCE

The women were asked for their contraceptive history and reasons for changes in the method used. In most cases this was straightforward, but some couples had at times used combined methods, e.g. sheath and safe period, and a few had a back-up method, e.g. if the wife ran out of pills the husband might use a sheath. Tables 5.2 and 5.3 give the contraception used by the couples in the 1951 and 1985 samples respectively, identifying all methods reportedly used in sequence.

Of the 57 couples in the earlier survey who used a male method first, 20 had chosen the sheath and 37 had used coitus interruptus (Table 5.2). Of the twelve wives who had initially taken responsibility nine used chemicals and three the diaphragm, the only ones in the sample to have used this method. Because the main methods available in the 1950s were disliked because they were 'messy' or interfered with sex, more couples had tried a combination of

TABLE 5.2

CONTRACEPTION USED IN SEQUENCE—1951 SAMPLE

First contraception used followed by any other(s) in sequence	No. of couples	
Diaphragm only	2	
Diaphragm–chemicals	1	
Chemicals only	7	12
Chemicals + safe period	1	
Chemicals–sheath	1	
Sheath only	14	
Sheath–coitus interruptus	1	
Sheath–chemicals + safe period	1	
Sheath–chemicals–coitus interruptus	1	20
Sheath–safe period	1	
Sheath + safe period	2	
Coitus interruptus only	35	
Coitus interruptus + chemicals	1	37
Coitus interruptus + safe period	1	
None used		90
Total		159

— = changed method
+ = combined methods

methods than in the recent sample. This usually meant trying to use the safe period alternating with another method.

In the 1985 study the pill had been the first choice of 139 of the 150 couples who had used contraception; of the remainder, eight started off using the sheath, but three soon changed to the pill, one wife used the diaphragm and two wives had a coil fitted (Table 5.3).

The new methods available to the 1985 couples were not without their problems. Some women had to give up taking the pill or had to have the coil removed for medical reasons. For example, five women developed conditions contraindicating the pill, namely high blood pressure, breast lumps, suspicious cervical smear, colitis and urinary tract infection. In addition, seven women came off the pill on account of side effects such as migraine, weight gain, depression and intermittent bleeding. Fears as a result of 'scares' about the pill (3 women) or apprehension after taking it for several years (9 women) had also led to discontinuation and this was sometimes the deciding factor in the timing of pregnancy. Two women had had to have a coil removed, one because of stomach cramps and one because of excessive bleeding.

TABLE 5.3

CONTRACEPTION USED IN SEQUENCE—1985 SAMPLE

First contraception used followed by any other(s) in sequence	*No. of couples*	
Pill only	93	
Pill–sheath	32[1]	
Pill–sheath + chemicals	1	
Pill–sheath-diaphragm	1	
Pill–sheath + safe period	2	
Pill–sheath–safe period	1	
Pill–diaphragm	4[1]	142
Pill–IUCD	5[2]	
Diaphragm + safe period	1	
Coil–pill–diaphragm	1	
Coil–pill–sheath	1	
Sheath only	5	
Sheath–pill	3	8
None used		8
Total		158

( ) returned to use pill
− = changed method
+ = combined methods

RESPONSIBILITY

The introduction of a widely acceptable new method for women had meant a dramatic change in overall responsibility for contraception (Table 5.4). Considering total experience of contraception, in 1951 nearly one-third of husbands had had sole responsibility, ten times as many as in 1985 when two-thirds of the wives had taken the full responsibility. Also one-quarter of couples in the recent study had used both male and female methods, a five-fold increase.

Considering only those couples in the 1951 sample who had ever used contraception, nearly three-quarters of husbands had been totally responsible (Table 5.4). One-sixth of wives had borne the responsibility using a variety of chemical preparations, the safe period and diaphragm, in order of popularity. For the remainder responsibility had been shared, most usually starting with a male method and changing to the less efficient female methods, e.g. sheath to safe period.

The situation in 1985 was quite different in that 70% of wives had been totally responsible for contraception, but only 3% of husbands (Table 5.4).

TABLE 5.4

RESPONSIBILITY FOR CONTRACEPTION

	Sample		Ever used contraception	
	1951	1985	1951	1985
(n)	(159)	(158)	(69)	(150)
Responsibility	%	%	%	%
Husband	31	3	73	3
Wife	7	66	16	70
Both	5	26	11	27
Neither	57	5	**	**
Total	100	100	100	100

The increase in couples who had shared responsibility partly reflects resort to the sheath if wives had had to come off the pill for health reasons, or if they followed medical advice to discontinue oral contraception some months prior to attempting conception.

SOURCE OF ADVICE AND SUPPLY

In the 1950s the Family Planning Clinic fitted nearly all diaphragms, only a few being fitted in exceptional circumstances by gynaecologists. All the three women in the earlier sample who used the diaphragm had attended the Clinic, as had four of the seven users in 1985, the remainder having been fitted by their general practitioner. The extent to which the GPs had become involved in family planning is shown by the fact that 101 of the 144 women in the 1985 sample who had used the pill had received prescriptions only from their GP, and a further 11 women had attended both the GP and the FPC; the remaining 32 women had received the pill only through the FPC. General practitioners had also fitted five of the seven women who used an IUCD.

CONTRACEPTIVE FAILURES

Table 5.5 gives the last method the women said they had used and indicates how many said they had still been using contraception when pregnancy occurred. In both studies, 'failures' were reported with all methods except for the diaphragm in 1951 and IUCD in 1985, but in each case only three couples were concerned. The unreliability of coitus interruptus is evident in that over half the users, all in the 1951 sample, reported failure.

Failures with the sheath were reported by one couple in 1951 and three couples in 1985. It is not always certain whether failures were genuinely due to the method, e.g. a burst sheath, or whether use was actually inconsistent, e.g. risks being taken if the husband had run out of supplies. There is some indication, however, that failures in 1985 were associated with use following

TABLE 5.5

LAST METHOD USED

	1951 No.	1985 No.
Coitus interruptus	37[21]	—
Sheath	15[1]	30[3]
Safe period	3[1]	2[1]
Chemicals only	10[1]	1
Combined methods	1[1]	1[1]
Diaphragm	3	6[1]
IUCD	Not available	3
Pill	Not available	107[1]
Total users	69[25]	150[7]

( ) Reported still using at conception

discontinuation of the pill, e.g. one woman advised to come off the pill after five years had resorted to the sheath and was 'very shocked' to have become pregnant 'after avoiding it for so long'. Women who followed medical recommendations to stop oral contraception and use an alternative for some months before they conceived usually chose the sheath and were unlikely to be particularly disconcerted if they became pregnant earlier than intended.

The safe period, as indicated earlier, was not always fully understood and the reported failure rate was high. Women attributed failure with combined methods to unsuccessful use of the safe period. Assuming this, two of the four women in 1951 and two of the three women in 1985 whose last method had been the safe period, said that it had let them down.

The messiness of chemical contraceptives was disliked and there was evidence of erratic use. Only one woman from the 1951 sample reported failure with the method. In the 1950s supplies were sometimes obtained from 'a pal at work' and as one woman reported, pregnancy had occurred when she had been sick and off work and, therefore, cut off from her source of supply.

Only one woman, who was in the recent sample, described failure of the diaphragm as 'the reason she was pregnant'. Initially, she had chosen the coil, but when this proved unsatisfactory she went on to oral contraception, but after several years was recommended 'to take a break' and when using the diaphragm she conceived. Apparently a few GPs still advise women to come off the pill from time to time in order to restore normal menstruation.

The only woman who reported failure with the pill, would not elaborate, merely repeating that 'it didn't suit her'.

PLANNING OF PREGNANCY

The women were asked why they had stopped using contraception if indeed they had done so. Table 5.6 shows that twice as many in the current sample

TABLE 5.6

PLANNING OF PREGNANCY BY CONTRACEPTION USERS

	1951	1985
(n)	(69)	(150)
Contraception		
Stopped		
to become pregnant	41	82
medical reasons	—	4
other factors	6	7
Uncertain use	17	3
Still using	36	4
Total users	100	100

reported stopping in order to become pregnant (82% compared with 41% in 1951). Medical reasons for coming off the pill or having an IUCD removed precipitated the decision for 4% of the 1985 sample. Some couples in both surveys had stopped using contraception for a variety of reasons, not necessarily wanting a pregnancy, but prepared to take the risk—these women sometimes reported that they got 'fed up' with using contraception or that some event such as moving house or going on holiday had disrupted their routine.

In each sample there were some women about whom it was uncertain whether or not they had been taking precautions. These were the erratic contraceptive users (17% in 1951 and 3% in 1985) who took chances. In the recent study they included women who were forgetful and found the discipline of taking the pill tiresome.

Nine times as many women in the 1951 as in the 1985 sample said that they had still been using contraception and trying to avoid pregnancy when it occurred (36% and 4% respectively). The details have already been discussed with references to reported failures, the difference between the studies being due to the unreliability of coitus interruptus.

Family Intentions

In the course of the AN interview, the primigravidae were asked about the sex of baby preferred, how many children they would like to have and the preferred interval between the first and the second. This information, however, was not asked of the initial quarter of the 1951 sample.

The 1951 women questioned were fairly equally divided between those who wanted a boy, wanted a girl or did not mind; whereas nearly half the husbands, a significantly high proportion, were said to want a boy (Table

TABLE 5.7

PREFERENCE FOR BOY OR GIRL

	1951*		1985†	
	Wife	*Husband*	*Wife*	*Husband*
(n)	(161)	(127)	(155)	(155)
Preference	%	%	%	%
Boy	32	49	15	23
Girl	33	34	12	10
None	35	17	73	67
Total	100	100	100	100

Wife v husband 1951 v 1985	$\lambda^2_{(2)} = 13.31$ $p \leqslant 0.001$	$\lambda^2_{(2)} = 3.94$ NS
Wife v wife	$\lambda^2_{(2)} = 45.96$ $p \leqslant 0.001$	
Husband v husband	$\lambda^2_{(2)} = 72.74$ $p \leqslant 0.001$	

* Excluding no data
† 2 knew sex from scanning. 1 seen postnatally only

5.7). The situation was quite changed by 1985 when the majority of women said that neither they nor their husbands had any sex preference for their first child, and although more husbands than wives wished for a boy, the difference was not statistically significant. This change over time away from a preferred sex to 'not minding' was highly significant for both the wives and husbands. A new feature was that two women in the 1985 sample already knew the sex of their baby as a result of scanning.

There was a significant difference in how many children the primigravidae in the two samples said they wanted to have (Table 5.8). The recent sample favoured smaller families, but more of the women were uncertain and less likely to be precise about numbers, wanting to wait and see how they got on before committing themselves. However, over half in both samples wanted 'two' or 'two or three' children.

Women who said that they wanted more than one child (except those who were expecting twins), were asked how long they would like before their second child was born. Although the most popular interval was 2 to 3 years in both samples, there had been a highly significant change to a shorter interval or uncertainty (Table 5.9). Whereas over one-third of the primigravidae in the earlier sample wanted at least three years before their second child, this applied to only half as many in the present sample.

As far as contraception was concerned, the knowledge, experience and attitudes of the married primigravidae in the two samples were vastly

TABLE 5.8

WIFE—NUMBER OF CHILDREN WANTED

	1951	1985
(n)	(151)*	(157)†
No. of children		
wanted	%	%
1	10	11
1-2	4	13
2	40	34
2-3	17	22
3	12	7
3-4	9	5
4+	5	1
Uncertain	3	7
Total	100	100

$$\lambda^2_{(7)} = 17.77 \quad p \leqslant 0.01$$

* Excluding no data
† 1 seen postnatally only

TABLE 5.9

WIFE—YEARS PREFERRED BETWEEN FIRST AND SECOND BABY

	1951	1985
(n)*	(127)	(137)
Years between	%	%
-2	12	30
2-3	49	41
3-4	20	14
4-5	8	2
5+	6	1
No preference	5	12
Total	100	100

$$\lambda^2_{(5)} = 26.23 \quad p \leqslant 0.001$$

* Excluding expecting twins, wanted only 1 child and no data

different. In general, fatalism had given way to acceptance that fertility could be controlled. The availability of the pill had transformed the situation and the initiative and responsibility for family planning now rested with wives and not husbands. Couples in the recent study emphasised their wish for a normal, healthy baby rather than one of a particular sex. Although a family of two children remained the most popular, the 1985 women tended to favour having fewer children, spaced nearer together.

## CHAPTER 6

Work Experience and Social Activities

Details of occupations are important in determining not only the socio-economic status achieved by the couple, but also the background and organisation of family life. Also in the early 1950s the significance of women continuing in employment during pregnancy was a matter of concern and special investigation (Illsley *et al.*, 1954). There was interest in the extent to which pregnancy interfered with a woman's everyday life and in particular any changes in her usual physical activity. This led to enquiries about recreation and social life.

Working Experience and Occupations

There were some important differences in the occupational experience of the two samples. The 1951 sample had lived through a war and nearly three-quarters of the men and one-tenth of the women had served in the Armed Forces and a few others had been conscripted to work of national importance. Moreover, as reported in Chapter 3, the school leaving age had been raised in the intervening years and opportunities for higher education had considerably increased. By 1985 the exploitation of North Sea oil had provided a dynamic impetus to the area economy which defied national trends in certain respects. Employment levels fell between the 1971 and 1981 censuses in Great Britain as a whole by about 4%, whereas in the Aberdeen area employment grew by nearly 19% (Bonney, 1986). The number of males in employment increased by 12% compared to a 9% national decline and that of females in employment increased by 28% compared to 5% nationally.

In both studies the women were asked about their own and their husband's occupational histories and these will be considered separately.

HUSBAND

Although husbands in the two samples were similar in age those in 1985 had had a shorter working life because of increased education and training; half had worked for less than ten years compared with one-third of the 1951 husbands ($p \leqslant 0.01$). Nevertheless, nearly twice as many husbands in 1985 had had at least five jobs (Table 6.1). Two jobs would have been the mode in both samples, but for the fact that most men in the 1951 sample had served in the Armed Forces which has been counted as a job. If after being demobbed a man returned to his previous employment, this has been taken as continuous employment. The difference in the number of jobs held by the husbands in the two samples is highly significant (Table 6.1).

Time in the present job (or period of unemployment) when the wife attended the ANC was similar between the two samples—nearly one-in-four of the husbands had held the job for less than a year, while one-in-twenty had been in the same job for at least ten years.

The husband's occupations have been divided in accordance with the Registrar General's Social Classification, but amalgamated into three

TABLE 6.1

HUSBAND—NUMBER OF JOBS

	1951	1985
(n)*	(187)	(157)
No. of Jobs	%	%
1	12	11
2	10	27
3	44	23
4	20	14
5	5	9
6+	9	16
Total	100	100

$$\lambda^2_{(5)} = 33.09 \quad p \leqslant 0.001$$

* Excluding not stated

TABLE 6.2

HUSBAND'S OCCUPATION

	Main before marriage		At booking	
	1951	1985	1951	1985
(n)	(213)	(158)	(213)	(158)
Occupations	%	%	%	%
Non manual	19	37	18	43
Skilled manual	46⎫ 51	43⎫ 45	46⎫ 51	39⎫ 40
Armed Forces	5⎭	2⎭	5⎭	1⎭
Other manual	30	18	31	17
Total	100	100	100	100

$$\lambda^2_{(2)} = 17.34 \quad p \leqslant 0.001 \qquad \lambda^2_{(2)} = 28.63 \quad p \leqslant 0.001$$

groups—non-manual (SC I, II and III non-manual), skilled manual (SC III remainder) and other manual (SC IV and V). Table 6.2 shows that over the years there had been a significant change in the husbands' employment in favour of non-manual occupations. For present purposes students have been included as non-manual workers as all were engaged in professional training. Men in the Armed Forces have been taken as skilled manual as all were working as drivers, fitters, etc. It will be noted that there was virtually no difference in the distribution of the husbands'occupation in the earlier sample between the main job before marriage and at the wife's booking, whereas the greater interval between marriage and booking in the recent study had allowed some occupational advancement.

The significant impact of North Sea oil development on employment in Aberdeen is demonstrated by the fact that one-third of the 1985 husbands were directly (18%) or indirectly (16%) employed in the industry. Antenatally, one-in-nine husbands worked off-shore on the oil rigs alternating two or three weeks away with a similar period at home.

The majority of husbands in both samples worked regular daytime hours (71% in 1951; 68% in 1985) and a further 11% did shift work. The remainder had variable working arrangements usually involving periods away from home according to contract requirements, e.g. construction workers or merchant seamen as well as oil rig workers in 1985. Nine husbands in 1951, but only one in 1985, were in the Armed Forces during their wife's pregnancy.

WIVES

Like the husbands, the wives in 1985 had worked for a shorter time than those in 1951 ($p \leqslant 0.05$) twice as many having worked for less than five years (15% compared with 7% in 1951). All women in the recent sample had been out to work whereas two women (one of whom was disabled) in the earlier sample had never been employed.

The work histories of the 1951 sample had been less affected by the war than those of their husbands. There was no significant difference either in the number of jobs the women had had (10% in each sample had had six or more) or in the time the women had spent in their present or last job although more of the 1951 sample had held this for less than a year (32% compared with 23% in 1985) reflecting the attitude to married women working at that time.

In the early 1950s it was customary in some occupations, e.g. teaching, for women to cease work on marriage, but in addition the policy of some firms (e.g. the Northern Co-operative Society) not to employ married women meant that women were obliged to leave when they married, and opportunities for temporary work were negligible. In the mid 1980s women were legally protected from such discrimination (Maternity Alliance, 1981) and marriage per se had not affected employment.

The Registrar General's Classification of Occupations is not entirely appropriate to women's occupations and for present purposes the occupations of the wives have been divided into three groups—professional, technical and clerical; distributive and skilled manual; other manual. Table 6.3 gives the women's main occupation before marriage and shows the highly significant increase in professional, technical and clerical occupations in 1985 and a particularly marked decline in other manual work compared with 1951.

There was a major difference between the samples in how many of the primigravidae worked during pregnancy and for how long. Nearly half the 1951 women had stopped work before they attended the ANC compared with one-tenth in 1985 (Table 6.3) although the recent sample attended later. Not only did more of the 1985 primigravidae work, but they continued significantly longer into pregnancy (Table 6.4). By 26 weeks gestation, 78% of the 1951 women were not in employment compared with 32% in 1985. Of women who worked during pregnancy, those in the 1951 sample stopped work on average at 20.5 weeks gestation compared with 25.6 weeks in the recent study ($t = 5.71$ $p \leqslant 0.001$). In both studies most women who worked during pregnancy did so full-time (88% in 1951; 92% in 1985).

The majority of women who worked cited pregnancy as the reason for leaving (89% in 1951; 78% in 1985). Medical reasons were nearly three times as frequent in 1985 (17% compared with 6% in 1951) and the conditions more varied. This does not necessarily imply that the 1985 sample had more problems given that they worked longer in pregnancy. The 1951 women had stopped work on account of lumbago, phlebitis, depression and a heart condition. In 1985 the medical reasons given included threatened abortion, excessive nausea, water retention, raised blood pressure, urinary tract infection, backache and exhaustion. In each study, a few women gave miscellaneous reasons, e.g. to care for a sick relative; contract ended; moved to Aberdeen.

A few women in both samples intended to carry on working throughout pregnancy. Two women in 1951 worked in the family shop and did piece work at home respectively. Of the six women in 1985, four were self-

TABLE 6.3

WIFE'S OCCUPATION

(n)	Main before marriage		At booking	
	1951	1985	1951	1985
	(213)	(158)	(213)	(158)
Occupation	%	%	%	%
Professional, technical and clerical	30	72	16	64
Distributive and skilled manual	41	21	17	20
Other manual	28	7	18	6
Not working	1	—	49	10
Total	100	100	100	100

$\lambda^2_{(2)} = 65.67$ $p \leqslant 0.001$ $\qquad$ $\lambda^2_{(2)} = 47.27$ $p \leqslant 0.001$

TABLE 6.4

DURATION OF PAID WORK DURING PREGNANCY

	1951	1985
(n)	(213)	(158)
Work—completed weeks		
gestation	%	%
0	36	8
10 or less	9	3
11–20	20	8
21–25	13	13
26–30	14	49
31 +	5	15
Continued working	1	4
Uncertain	2	—
Total	100	100

No paid work during pregnancy v Rest $\lambda^2_{(1)} = 21.24$ $p \leqslant 0.001$

employed, e.g. typist and craft worker, and two only did a few hours sessional work a week. All these women had flexible working arrangements under their own control.

Social Activities

A major factor affecting the social activities of the 1985 sample compared with the 1951 was the use of a car. In the early 1950s cars were owned mainly by couples when the husband was in a professional occupation and some went with the man's job, e.g. commercial travelling. A routine question about ownership or use of a car was never considered in the earlier study, but 6% of the sample were known to have one. In contrast, 73% of the 1985 couples had a car they either owned or were provided with by the husband's firm and a further 3% had the use of a relative's car. Having a car greatly facilitated their opportunities for visiting and outings of all kinds.

Opportunities for sports and recreation had been transformed between the studies precipitated in the 1970s as the oil industry developed. In the early 1950s there were two public swimming baths, the older of which had to be closed down, a skating rink which later closed and golf courses. Adult sports tended to be based on colleges, the University and a few firms or organisations; there were some tennis and bowling clubs and some churches provided facilities, e.g. badminton. However, dance halls were almost universally popular until a couple began 'going steady'.

By 1985 sports and recreational facilities had mushroomed providing for a wider range of activities in different settings. There were numerous swimming pools in schools as well as in hotels and clubs which often provided saunas and squash courts. Discos, like the earlier dance halls, were popular before marriage. A plethora of restaurants and bars, no longer able to exclude women, encouraged social meetings and eating out. Not found in 1985 was the attitude fairly prevalent in the early 1950s that a pregnant woman was a public embarrassment which kept some women within the confines of their home, avoiding daytime or public outings as far as possible.

Nearly half the 1985 primigravidae reported taking part in some sport or physical recreation about the time they became pregnant, three times as many as in the 1951 sample (46% compared with 15% in 1951). Most of the 1951 women only mentioned dancing which they had given up early in pregnancy; the remainder had stopped badminton, cycling, skating, swimming or tennis.

Swimming was the most popular sport of the 1985 primigravidae—16 women continued to swim during pregnancy; two started swimming and 21 gave it up. Keepfit classes attracted two new recruits, two continued during pregnancy and 16 had stopped attending soon after they became pregnant. A more varied list of other sports discontinued during pregnancy included horseriding, jogging, squash and volleyball in addition to badminton, cycling, tennis and dancing.

The majority of women in both samples had passive recreations, e.g. knitting, while TV and videos, commonplace in the lives of the 1985 primigravidae were unknown in the 1950s when cinema going was popular.

In summary, compared with the 1951 sample, the 1985 couples were more likely to be non-manual workers and more worked during pregnancy and continued longer. Women in the recent sample were also more likely to have recreational interests outside their homes, including sports and physical activities of all kinds.

## CHAPTER 7

Attitude to and Experience of Pregnancy and Childbirth

The women in the two samples were facing their first pregnancy in different social and medical situations. In the 1950s there was relatively little general discussion of pregnancy and labour and few visual aids; most information was gathered from relatives and friends. Some of the mothers of the 1951 primigravidae had had domiciliary confinements and were not always encouraging about their daughters going into hospital and 'all the fuss'. In contrast, the 1985 primigravidae through the mass media had had numerous opportunities to see films, to hear discussions and to read articles on every aspect of pregnancy and childbirth. They were only too aware of the medicalisation of childbirth and some were sophisticated about the controversy surrounding it. Given these differences how did the primigravidae, 34 years apart, differ in their approach to experiences of childbearing?

Information on attitudes, intentions and experiences were obtained at the ANC and postnatal home interviews. Details on obstetric experience was available from data routinely recorded in the computerised Aberdeen Maternity and Neonatal Data Bank.

Antenatal

ANTENATAL CARE

More of the 1951 primigravidae attended the ANC early and late compared with primigravidae in 1985 (Table 7.1). The difference in timing is partly explained by the booking procedures. In 1951 the women attended the clinic when they chose in order to have the pregnancy confirmed, whereas in 1985 they first went to their general practitioner and in response to a referral the hospital sent them an appointment to attend the ANC. Thus, not surprisingly, relatively few women in 1985 had attended before 11 weeks. In both studies, however, about two-thirds of the women had attended by 16 weeks gestation. The high proportion of relatively late attenders in 1951 reflects the higher rate of prenuptial conception as it was customary to delay the first visit to the clinic until after marriage (Illsley, 1956a; b).

TABLE 7.1

GESTATION AT FIRST ANTENATAL CLINIC ATTENDANCE
CUMULATIVE PERCENTAGE

	1951	1985
(n)	(213)	(158)
Gestation—completed weeks	%	%
10 or less	25	6
11–15	66	71
16–20	87	96
21 or more	100	100

$$\lambda_{(3)}^{2} = 38.82 \quad p \leqslant 0.001$$

ANTENATAL CLASSES

The provision of classes was very different at the time of the two studies. In 1951 the dietitians and social workers combined to give talks on eating during pregnancy, welfare foods and insurance requirements for maternity benefits; these were given each week and the women could choose when to attend. Only one-quarter of the women attended, but nurses and social workers routinely gave information about welfare foods and benefits to each woman individually. About a month before their expected date of delivery the women were invited to attend a talk and demonstration on the process of labour given by a consultant obstetrician. Again, the women showed relatively little interest, and although 59% said that they were going to attend only 38% did so. This poor attendance reflected the fatalism of many in the earlier sample, nearly one-in-eight of women adamantly refused to think about labour.

The situation for the 1985 primigravidae was different in that they were offered a course of classes under the aegis of the Health Education Department of the Grampian Health Board. The classes, some of which were also for husbands, extended over eight weeks. They were taught by health visitors and took place in clinics and health centres. The classes provided information about pregnancy, labour, delivery and mothercraft as well as instruction in prophylactic exercises. Primigravidae were invited to attend from about 32 weeks. Altogether, 85% of the current sample attended at least part of the course and many went to all the classes. The extent to which the 1985 women found these classes helpful is reported in the Appendix.

HUSBAND'S ATTITUDES

Reporting what their husbands had said, the great majority of wives in each sample said that they were pleased about the pregnancy and looking forward to becoming fathers (83% in 1951 and 96% in 1985). In 1951 ten husbands were reported to be indifferent and eight to have negative attitudes—the wives described these husbands as being jealous or not liking babies. One husband, married during the pregnancy, was said to be very hostile to the prospect of fatherhood and he later denied paternity. The attitudes of the remaining ten 1951 husbands could not be classified, either because they worked away and the wife was unsure how they felt, or because the wife reported that 'they just wished it was all over'. One husband wanted only a boy.

Husbands in 1951 kept a low profile in the background, whereas in 1985 they were encouraged to take an active part by attending some classes along with their wives, and by being present at the confinement. No husband was said to resent the pregnancy although some indifference was attributed to three husbands who were said to be reticent characters. Four wives, two of whom had married during pregnancy, reported that their husbands were slow at showing interest.

Labour and Delivery

AGE AT DELIVERY

The women and to a lesser extent their husbands, were significantly older in 1985 than in 1951 (Table 7.2). Mean ages had increased from 23.9 to 25.5 years for the women and from 26.6 to 27.9 for their husbands. There were over six times as many teenagers in 1951, but only half as many women in their late twenties. In the earlier sample more than half the women were in their early twenties when they had their first baby. As for the husbands, nearly twice as many were aged under 25 in 1951 as in 1985.

TABLE 7.2

AGE AT DELIVERY

	Wife		Husband	
	1951	1985	1951	1985
(n)	(213)	(158)	(213)	(158)
Age	%	%	%	%
–19	13	2	2	1
20–24	52	41	39	21
25–29	24	46	36	46
30–34	8	10	15	23
35+	3	1	8	9
Total	100	100	100	100

$$\lambda_{(4)}^2 = 31.10 \quad p \leqslant 0.001 \qquad \lambda_{(4)}^2 = 14.86 \quad p \leqslant 0.01$$

TABLE 7.3

GESTATION AT DELIVERY
CUMULATIVE PERCENTAGE

(n)	1951 (213)	1985 (158)
Completed weeks of gestation	%	%
36 or less	8	8
37	16	11
38	26	24
39	48	46
40	77	79
41	91	99
42 or over	100	100
	$\lambda^2_{(4)} = 15.92 \; p \leqslant 0.01$	

GESTATION

The mean length of gestation was similar in the two samples (39.1 and 39.2 completed weeks). There were, however, some significant differences in the distributions (Table 7.3). Fewer of the 1985 primigravidae gave birth after 42 weeks, reflecting the policy of induction developed as the potential hazards of postmaturity were established. Changes in obstetric management may also have accounted for the fall in very premature deliveries (32 weeks or less) in the recent sample (1.3% compared with 3.3% in 1951), although overall the proportions of births at 36 weeks of gestation or less were similar.

INDUCTION OF LABOUR

It was to be expected in view of the well known changes in obstetric practice that significantly more women in the 1985 sample would have labour induced (Table 7.4). The onset of labour had been spontaneous for 84% of the 1951 sample, but this applied to only 59% in 1985. In the 1951 sample induction was by artificial rupture of membranes (ARM), syntocin drip or more rarely a combination of the two. In 1985, although the incidence of ARM had increased it was usually combined with the administration of syntocin. For 9% of the 1985 women the onset of labour followed the insertion of a prostin pessary to ripen the cervix, a method not available in 1951. Also in the recent study, obstetricians had elected that five women should be delivered by CS on account of medical or anticipated obstetric problems, and three of these were carried out before 36 weeks.

TABLE 7.4

INDUCTION OF LABOUR AND METHOD

	1951	1985
(n)	(213)	(158)
Labour	%	%
Not induced	84	59
Induced by		
ARM	8	4
Syntocin	5	6
ARM and syntocin	3	19
Prostin pessary	—	9
Elective caesarean section	—	3
Total	100	100

Not induced v induced $\lambda^2_{(1)} = 26.86$ $p \leqslant 0.001$

COMPLICATIONS

Certain complications of labour and delivery showed marked increases in the 1985 sample (Table 7.5). In some cases more frequent or detailed examination may be involved as the increased use of technology, e.g. electronic fetal monitors, facilitated the early identification of possible problems or abnormalities. This particularly affected the diagnosis of fetal distress which appeared to have increased over four-fold, apparently affecting the majority of babies in the recent sample. The broad classification used by the obstetricians made no allowance for the usual variability in fetal blood pressure and has now been discontinued.

The coding of pre-eclamptic toxaemia (PE) in the Data Bank was based on definitions and gradings laid down by Nelson (1955). In 1985 one-third of the sample were recorded as having hypertension/mild PE, over 60%

TABLE 7.5

PERCENT OF SAMPLE WITH COMPLICATIONS OF LABOUR AND DELIVERY

	1951	1985
(n)	(213)	(158)
Complication	*% of sample*	*% of sample*
Hypertension/mild PE	19	33
Moderate or severe PE	8	11
Antepartum haemorrhage	4	15
Episiotomy	35	57
Fetal distress	18	83
Postpartum haemorrhage	11	3

increase, and the proportion with moderate or severe PE was nearly 50% higher. Antepartum haemorrhage was recorded for one in seven of the recent sample, nearly four times as many as in 1951. About one-third of the women in the earlier sample had had an episiotomy. In later years this became so routine that for a time it was no longer coded in the Data Bank— but as time went on moderation prevailed and in the 1985 sample, 57% had had an episiotomy. Another major complication was postpartum haemorrhage affecting over three times as many women in 1951 as in the later survey, the decline in its incidence reflecting the routine of giving oxytocics (Lancet, 1986). However, one 1985 woman was given a blood transfusion following primary postpartum haemorrhage. One woman in each sample had a retained placenta and in 1951 one woman needed a cervical repair.

METHOD OF DELIVERY

As anticipated, fewer of the 1985 sample had had a spontaneous delivery (Table 7.6). The proportion delivered by forceps (34%) had almost doubled and that by CS (12%) had increased six fold. The relatively small proportion of assisted breech deliveries had declined. Of the three sets of twins in the earlier sample, two sets had been delivered spontaneously and in the third set one baby, a breech, had had an assisted delivery. In the recent sample one set of twins was delivered spontaneously and one set by CS.

PAIN RELIEF AND ANALGESICS

It was exceptional for the 1985 women not to have received help in bearing the pain of labour and delivery (Table 7.7) and often they had used more than one method. In marked contrast over one-third of the 1951 sample according to the records had received no pain relievers or anaesthetics, but

TABLE 7.6

METHOD OF DELIVERY
(excluding twins)

(n)	1951 (210)	1985 (156)
Method of Delivery	%	%
Spontaneous	76	52
Forceps	19	34
Breech	3	2
Caesarean section	2	12
Total	100	100

$$\lambda_{(3)}^2 = 32.09 \quad p \leqslant 0.001$$

TABLE 7.7

METHOD OF PAIN RELIEF AND ANAESTHESIA

	1951	1985
(n)	(213)	(158)
Method	%	%
	of sample	of sample
None	37	4
Gas and air	29	51
Pethidine	11	63
Epidural	3	44
General anaesthetic*	19	6†
Other	18	6

* Additionally after delivery on account of complications 2% in each sample

† One woman included here had two general anaesthetics—for a caesarean section and postnatally

the use of gas and air may not always have been noted. Whereas, in 1951 all breech and nearly all forceps deliveries were carried out under general anaesthetic, in 1985 the majority were done under an epidural. Pethidine had been given to some women who had forceps deliveries, but one woman in 1985 had only had gas and air. Three of the four CSs in 1951 had been done under an epidural compared with nine of the 19 CSs in 1985. A general anaesthetic had been given for the remaining CSs, although three of the nine women involved had initially been given an epidural for pain relief.

More women in 1951 had received 'other' methods of pain relief (Table 7.7), usually sedatives; however, eight women in 1951 had had morphia. Six women in 1985 had used the pulsar which was introduced to AMH while the study was in progress. Due to complications (e.g. retained products of conception), five women in 1951 and three in 1985 had a general anaesthetic postnatally.

HUSBAND'S PARTICIPATION

A major difference between the two studies was in the encouragement and opportunities given to husbands to be present in the labour ward. No husband in the 1951 sample attended his wife's confinement, whereas it was exceptional for the 1985 husbands not to be there (4.7%). Most husbands in 1985 were present throughout labour and delivery; for medical or personal reasons 7% were present during labour but not when the baby was born, whereas 2% of husbands only arrived in time for the delivery. The attitudes and experiences of the couples are reported in the Appendix.

The 1985 woman and their husbands were older when they had their first child. Significant differences in the time the women attended the ANC could be accounted for by changes in procedure increasing the involvement of GPs and by changes in social behaviour reducing prenuptial conception. The 1985 women took more advantage of antenatal classes provided than did their fatalistic 1951 counterparts and the greater involvement of husbands has been revolutionary. The recent sample experienced more obstetric interference—significantly more had labour induced so that fewer babies were 'postmature'; more had operative deliveries and more were given pain relievers and anaesthesia: also more of them experienced all complications except postpartum haemorrhage compared with women in the earlier sample.

## CHAPTER 8

Outcome and Postnatal Experience

The outcome of pregnancies for these primigravidae 34 years apart was remarkably similar—in 1951, 96.3% had a singleton baby who survived, compared with 96.8% in 1985 (Table 8.1). The proportions of stillbirths, later deaths and twins were also similar. Although the perinatal mortality rate (PMR) was lower in the 1985 sample, 18.8 compared with 27.8 (per 1,000 births) in the 1951 sample and for singletons only 19.2 compared with 23.8 respectively, the differences were not statistically significant. However, significant reductions had occurred in the PMR for all Aberdeen first births

TABLE 8.1

OUTCOME OF PREGNANCY

	1951		1985	
	No.	%	No.	%
Singleton				
Livebirth—survived	205	96.3	153	96.8
—died	2	0.9	1	0.6
Stillbirth	3	1.4	2	1.3
Twins				
Both survived	2	0.9	2	1.3
1 survived, 1 died	1	0.5	—	—
Total	213	100.0	158	100.0

irrespective of marital status and pregnancy number (Table 8.2). In each study, the PMR for the sample was not significantly different from the overall PMR in the three different marital status and pregnancy number populations. It must be concluded that by chance the PMR in the 1951 sample was lower than expected while that in the 1985 sample was higher giving a non-significant difference. This applied for singletons and also overall, including multiple births. Because of the special problems associated with twins and their care, the following analysis will concentrate on singletons.

TABLE 8.2

PERINATAL MORTALITY RATES (PER 1000 TOTAL BIRTHS) IN
PRIMIPARAE FOR DIFFERENT POPULATIONS BY MARITAL STATUS AND
PREGNANCY NUMBER

	Singletons			All births		
	1951	1985		1951	1985	
Study sample Subgroup of all Aberdeen primiparae	23.8	19.2	NS	27.8	18.8	NS
Married 1st pregnancy only	39.3	12.1	****	40.9	11.9	****
All married	37.0	11.8	****	38.9	15.0	****
All primiparae	38.0	15.5	****	40.0	17.7	****

****p ⩽ 0.001

Singletons

SEX

Over half the singletons were boys as might be expected, but there were
rather more boys in 1985—55% compared with 51% in 1951. A similar
proportion of mothers in both studies had a baby of the sex for which they
had expressed a preference when interviewed antenatally (47% in 1951; 44%
in 1985).

BIRTHWEIGHT

The distribution of singleton birthweights were very similar between the two
samples. Low birthweight (LBW) babies, i.e. those weighing less than 2500g,
accounted for 9% in 1951 and 8% in 1985 (Table 8.3). Mean birthweights
were little changed from 3197g in 1951 to 3205g in 1985.

DEATHS

With the exception of one stillbirth in 1951 attributed to asphyxia and one
death during surgery for a congenital heart defect in 1985, deaths occurred
amongst low birthweight babies. The other two stillbirths in 1951 were due
to tertiary tear with internal haemorrhage and to 'prematurity', i.e. LBW
and short gestation; the two in 1985 were due to cardiac failure with
placental infarction and to rhesus isoimmunisation. The deaths in 1951 were
attributed to multiple congenital malformations incompatible with survival
and to 'prematurity'—the babies lived for 1 hour and 6 days respectively.

TABLE 8.3

BIRTHWEIGHT OF SINGLETONS

	1951		1985	
Birthweight (g)	*No.*	*%*	*No.*	*%*
Less than 2500	19[4]	9	12[2]	8
2500-2999	39	19	35[1]	22
3000-3499	96[1]	46	74	48
3500-3999	47	22	28	18
4000 or over	9	4	7	4
Total	210[5]	100	156[3]	100
	$\lambda_{(4)}^2 = 1.78$ Not significant			
Mean (g)	3197 ± 506		3205 ± 508	
	$t = 0.14$ Not significant			

( ) Stillbirths and deaths

CONDITION AT BIRTH

The ways in which the physical condition of the baby was assessed in the two studies were different and, therefore, the results are not directly comparable. In 1951 a subjective grading A to E was made soon after birth whereas in 1985 Apgar scores were used (Table 8.4).

In the 1951 sample, two-thirds of babies were classed as in very good condition (A) and a further one-fifth as good (B). Of the five who were rated poor (D), three were LBW babies of whom two died and the other spent 16 days in the Special Nursery. Low birthweight was not incompatible with a good grading, as seven of the 17 LBW babies were reckoned to be in very good condition.

In the recent sample, nine out of ten babies achieved an Apgar score of 9

TABLE 8.4

CONDITION OF BABIES AT BIRTH—LIVEBORN SINGLETONS ONLY

	1951			1985	
	No.	*%*		*No.*	*%*
Grade			*Apgar score at 5 minutes*		
A	137[7]	67	10	42[2]	27
B	40[2]	19	9	98[6]	64
C	25[5]	12	8	8[1]	5
D	5[3]	2	7 or less	6[1]	4
Total	207[17]	100		154[10]	100

( ) Less than 2500g, i.e. LBW

or 10 at five minutes; these included the baby who died subsequently during heart surgery. Again, the majority of LBW babies scored well.

However, with a few exceptions in 1951 all LBW babies were admitted to the Special Nursery although in some cases very briefly as a precautionary measure (Table 8.5). Not only were more of the 1951 babies admitted to the Special Nursery (20% compared with 13% in 1985), but they stayed in longer—8% being admitted for more than one week compared with 3% in 1985), which undoubtedly reflects the improved technology and facilities in neonatal care. In 1951 babies tended to be admitted for one or two days on account of respiratory distress or cyanotic attacks, though one suffered from excessive moulding of the head and one who had an oesophageal atresia was transferred to the Children's Hospital for operation. Somewhat longer stays were on account of thrush and other infections, facial palsy, haemolytic anaemia and scalp sinuses. A baby who suffered from erythroblastosis needed two blood transfusions and was in for 24 days. The longest stays were usually associated with preterm delivery and LBW; one baby was kept in for 31 days and another for 40 days.

The same pattern is seen in the reasons for the 1985 admissions to the Special Nursery. All LBW babies were routinely admitted for observation and half were kept there for only one day. Jaundice was recorded as the sole or a complementary reason why some babies were detained for several days; also one baby had Hirschsprung's disease. Thrush and facial palsy were not mentioned. The longest stay was 38 days for a preterm LBW baby who suffered from severe respiratory distress, hypoglycaemia and hypocalcaemia; the mother became depressed and was readmitted for 'bonding' one week prior to the baby's discharge.

Congenital anomalies and certain conditions requiring further check-up were noted for the 1985 babies—hypospadias, hydrocele, undescended testicles (2), metatarsus varus, pigmented naevi (2) and a systolic heart

TABLE 8.5

SPECIAL NURSERY ADMISSIONS—LIVEBORN SINGLETONS ONLY

	1951		1985	
No. of days	No.	%	No.	%
0	165[3]	80	134	87
1	*3[1]	2	7[5]	4
2	†11[1]	5	†5[1]	3
3–7	*11[1]	5	4	3
8–14	8[4]	4	3[3]	2
15 or over	9[7]	4	1[1]	1
Total	207[17]	100	154[10]	100

* 1 died at AMH
† 1 transferred to Children's Hospital for surgery
( ) Less than 2500g i.e. LBW

murmur. This reflects the routine paediatric checks and the follow up of babies with certain conditions which only became established practice in the mid 1960s after major staffing changes and reorganisation of perinatal care.

Infant Feeding

In addition to the details in the obstetric records the women in both samples were asked at 13 weeks postnatally about their experiences in feeding the singleton babies while they were in AMH. For present purposes four feeding groups have been identified:

1. *Breast.* Mothers in this group were fully breast feeding on discharge.
2. *Complementary.* These mothers were unable to satisfy their babies and had to introduce some artificial feeding. The babies were receiving both breast and artificial feeding on discharge.
3. *Breast to artificial.* All these mothers had tried breast feeding, but had abandoned it sometimes after a trial with complementary feeding. All the babies went out of AMH fully artificially fed.
4. *Artificial.* These mothers never attempted breast feeding.

Table 8.6 shows that whereas only 1 in 50 babies were never put to the breast in 1951, this applied to 1 in 4 babies in 1985. Such a difference reflects the change in hospital policy on infant feeding in the intervening years. In 1951 women were expected to breast feed and put under pressure to do so. It was accepted that breast feeding was best for both the mother and the baby, and incidentally, that it was easier for the hospital staff, although this is open to question.

At the time there was a good deal of research going on into the size and development of breasts, the quantity and biochemical composition of breast milk, and feeding progress (Hytten, 1954; Hytten and MacQueen, 1954;

TABLE 8.6

INFANT FEEDING IN AMH—SURVIVING SINGLETONS ONLY

	(n)	1951 (205) %	1985 (153) %
1	Breast only	82	54
2	Complementary	7	7
3	Breast to artificial	9	13
4	Artificial only	2	26
	Total	100	100

$$\lambda_{(3)}^2 = 53.33 \quad p \leqslant 0.001$$

Hytten and Leitch, 1971). Obstetricians routinely checked the breasts and nipples of primigravidae and advised about care during pregnancy and about treatment to overcome potential problems such as inverted nipples. In 1985 the situation was completely changed as the women could choose how to feed their babies although any advice received or literature read would have encouraged breast feeding. Obstetricians, however, seldom examined breasts (Macintyre, 1978). In fact breast preparation in pregnancy has been reported to be of no value (Ingleman-Sundberg, 1958).

1. BREAST FEEDING GROUP

In 1951, 82% of the sample left AMH totally breast feeding their babies, compared with 54% of the 1985 sample. For the majority of these mothers breast feeding had been straightforward. However, more mothers in the recent survey had encountered problems (40% compared with 17% in 1951) and more babies had received occasional 'top-up' feeds (46% compared with 10% in 1951).

The main problems in both samples were difficulties with the baby fixing properly and delay in establishing an adequate supply of milk. Cracked or sore nipples were more frequent in 1985, but there may have been some under-recording in 1951. Of course, as sucking stimulates lactation anything which prevents a baby from fixing or sucking properly, e.g. inverted nipples or the baby being initially too weak to suckle, may inhibit lactation.

In 1951 'top-up' feeds were occasionally given if establishing lactation was difficult, or if the baby seemed to be constantly hungry; however, in one case it was to give an exhausted mother a night's rest. Similar problems had arisen for the 1985 mothers, but it is an indication of more flexible attitudes to feeding that 20 babies had been artificially fed for one or two nights in order to give the mothers undisturbed sleep.

2. COMPLEMENTARY FEEDING GROUP

The proportions of babies receiving both breast and artificial feeds on discharge were similar in the two samples, i.e. 7%. In 1951 complementary feeding was attributed to inadequate lactation per se, whereas in 1985 another reported cause was that babies (3) did not fix well and were slow feeders. In addition, two mothers did not appear to have had any problems with breast feeding, but preferred to have the babies artificially fed at night so that they could sleep.

3. BREAST TO ARTIFICIAL FEEDING GROUP

More mothers in 1985 had attempted breast feeding while in AMH, but given it up entirely before they were discharged (13% compared with 9% in 1951). All the mothers in 1951 had encountered problems, often inter-related difficulties with fixing, slow feeding, sore nipples and inadequate lactation. Some mothers soon gave up while others persevered. For example, when a baby had difficulty fixing on to mis-shapen nipples, one mother had to give complementary feeds as well as expressed breast milk, but as days went by without any improvement she reluctantly abandoned breast feeding. Babies sometimes became 'lazy' about suckling after being given a bottle feed, generating a vicious circle.

The 1985 mothers who gave up breast feeding had similar experiences, some readily giving up when any difficulty arose whereas others only gradually accepted artificial feeding. However, two women gave up because they did not enjoy breast feeding and another because she was concerned because she 'couldn't see what the baby was getting'. By contrast one woman whose milk was described as 'murky' was advised to give artificial feeds while a sample was sent for chemical analysis; as the baby was doing well on the bottle she decided not to revert to breast feeding even though the laboratory tests proved negative.

4. ARTIFICIAL FEEDING GROUP

In 1951 only 2% of mothers never attempted breast feeding compared with 26% in 1985. In the earlier study two mothers resisted the pressures and flatly refused to breast feed, another who had been treated for syphilis during pregnancy was advised not to do so, and a fourth whose baby was admitted to the Special Nursery had grossly inverted nipples and was reported never to have had any milk. In contrast the mothers who chose not to breast feed in 1985 had no inclination to do so and felt under no pressure from hospital staff. Only two gave contributory reasons, one having felt exhausted, and the other having had pyrexia of unknown origin.

EXPRESSING BREAST MILK

Over nine times as many mothers in 1985 had experience of expressing breast milk (47% compared with 5% in 1951). The most important cause for

TABLE 8.7

REASON BREAST MILK EXPRESSED—MOTHERS OF SURVIVING SINGLETONS ONLY

	1951 No.	1985 No.
Baby in Special Nursery/Children's Hospital	3	10
Problems with fixing or feeding	2	5
Problems with breasts or nipples	5	24
Convenience	—	9
For experience	—	4
For biochemical analysis	—	1
No. who expressed milk	10	53
% of those who attempted breast feeding	5.3	47
% of those discharged breast or complementary feeding	5.5	58

expressing in both samples was a problem with breast engorgement or cracked nipples, followed by the baby being in the Special Nursery or in the case of one baby in the Children's Hospital (Table 8.7). The only other reason in 1951 was a problem with fixing, which also featured in 1985. An additional feature in the present sample, however, was that some women had expressed milk for the nurses to give by bottle if necessary, while they slept during the night. A few had simply wanted to learn how to do it under supervision in case it should be necessary after they went home. Finally, as already indicated, one woman had expressed her 'murky' milk for analysis.

OVERALL PROBLEMS

In each period the identification of the problem(s) encountered by those who attempted breast feeding is based on the total information available. Thus, of the fewer mothers who breast fed in 1985, nearly twice as many are recorded as having problems (56% compared with 30% in 1951) and all types of problems had increased, except those specific to the baby's medical condition, i.e. 'other' (Table 8.8).

TABLE 8.8

PROBLEMS WITH BREAST FEEDING (BF) OR REASONS FOR GIVING UP—
MOTHERS OF SURVIVING SINGLETONS ONLY

	1951 (201) % of BF mothers	1985 (113) % of BF mothers
(No. of mothers who tried breast feeding)		
Baby—fixing	13	28
—slow feeder	2	9
—other	2	1
Mother—establishing lactation	15	17
—nipples	6	20
—engorgement	4	6
BF mothers with problem(s)	30	56

Problems in establishing lactation and difficulties with the baby fixing were of fairly similar importance in 1951 (15% and 13% respectively). However, in 1985 although the proportion of mothers who had difficulties with lactation was only slightly increased, the proportion of babies reported to have had difficulty in fixing was more than double and this was the most frequent cause of problems. To some extent such early problems may have reflected the increased use of anaesthetics and analgesics (Richards and Bernal, 1972), but also hospital staff were less experienced in helping mothers who wished to breast feed. Three times as many mothers were recorded as having problems with nipples, but there may have been some under-recording of sore as opposed to cracked nipples in the earlier sample. More babies in 1985 were said to have posed problems with feeding slowly and more women had had engorged breasts.

FEEDING GROUPS AND CERTAIN CHARACTERISTICS

In 1951 women who were fully breast feeding on discharge were most likely to have had a spontaneous delivery and not to have had a general anaesthetic. However, this did not apply in 1985 (Table 8.9).

In both studies, the breast feeding group contained the highest proportion of professional, technical and clerical workers. However, in 1985 the proportion is fairly similar in the three groups of mothers who had tried breast feeding, whereas considerably fewer mothers who had always artificially fed their babies were in these occupations.

The intentions the women expressed antenatally about feeding proved an important indicator of what they would actually do, especially in the recent study when they had a choice. However, despite the different policies on infant feeding at the times the studies were carried out, a fairly similar proportion of women in the two surveys had stated antenatally that they definitely wished to breast feed (54% in 1951 and 59% in 1985). However, more 1985 mothers were definite about wishing to bottle feed (19% compared with 6% in 1951). Women in the earlier study, knowing that they would virtually have no choice in the matter, were more likely to be equivocal or to say that they would give breast feeding 'a try' (33% compared with 10% in 1985). The remaining women vaguely favoured bottle feeding or had no preference. Table 8.9 shows the importance of attitudes as in 1985 no mother who had stated a definite preference for bottle feeding attempted to breast feed. Conversely, it was exceptional for a woman who had intended to breast feed not to try, and the great majority in all three breast feeding groups had expressed a definite intention to breast feed. In both studies the highest proportion of women with a positive attitude to breast feeding antenatally was in the complementary feeding group; although numbers were small, this indicates the way in which these women (and also some who changed to artificial feeding while in AMH) had persevered with breast feeding and struggled to overcome problems encountered. In 1951 a few women who had definitely wished to bottle feed nevertheless went out of hospital fully breast feeding.

PROBLEMS IN THE PUERPERIUM

Throughout the years conditions posing medical problems or requiring treatment in the puerperium have been coded routinely for analysis, but the procedure has changed. In 1951 it was done by medical staff, whereas in 1985 it was done by specially trained clerical staff under the strict supervision of consultant obstetricians.

About one-fifth of women in both samples were noted in the hospital records as having at least one problem complicating their postnatal recovery

TABLE 8.9

PERCENT IN EACH FEEDING GROUP WITH CERTAIN CHARACTERISTICS—SURVIVING SINGLETONS ONLY

	1951				1985			
	Breast	Comp.	Br. to A.	Art.	Breast	Comp.	Br. to A.	Art.
(n)	(168)	(15)	(18)	(4)	(82)	(11)	(20)	(40)
Spontaneous delivery	81	67	61	75	46	64	55	52
General anaesthetic	18	33	28	25	6	0	15	12
Professional/clerical occupation	31	27	17	25	79	73	70	57
AN intention re feeding								
Breast definite	54	69	61	0	80	82	75	2
Artificial definite	6	0	0	100	0	0	0	72
Uncertain	40	31	39	0	20	18	25	26

(Table 8.10). Some changes in emphasis are readily explicable in terms of changing obstetric or infant feeding practices, e.g. fewer problems with genital and perineal sepsis, but more with abdominal (CS) wound infections in 1985; more breast problems in 1951 when virtually all the women started breast feeding. In 1985 three women suffered dural taps following an epidural and two complained of the side effects of hemineverin; in contrast only one woman in 1951 was reported to have suffered as a result of treatment—and she had been given a combination of heroin and sedatives from which she took time to recover and the baby was narcotised. There would appear to have been an increase in secondary postpartum haemorrhage requiring dilatation and curettage (D and C) for retained products of conception. Two women in the earlier sample were readmitted for D and C, as were three in 1985 one of whom developed septicaemia; in addition, one woman had been treated while still in AMH and had been given a blood transfusion. (Another woman in 1985 had also had a blood transfusion after suffering a primary postpartum haemorrhage, as reported in Chapter 7).

TABLE 8.10

RECORDED PROBLEMS IN THE PUERPERIUM—MOTHERS OF SURVIVING SINGLETONS ONLY

(n)	1951 (205)	1985 (153)
Infections—active TB	1†	—
respiratory	4	1
urinary tract	17	7
Pyrexia of unknown origin	3†	4
Sepsis—genital	9†	2
abdominal wound	—	4
Anaemia	3	2
Effects of medication/anaesthetic—dural tap	—	3
other	1	—
Persistent raised blood pressure	1	2
Deep vein thrombosis	1	—
Superficial phlebitis	1	—
Breast engorgement/mastitis	7	1
Secondary PPH—in AMH	—	1
readmitted	2	3
Arcuate uterus	1	—
Depression	—	1
No. with problem(s)	43	31
No. with no problem	162	122
% with problem(s)	21.0	20.3

† One woman transferred to City Hospital

When interviewed postnatally, eight women in the 1985 sample reported extra problems, and a further 18 women described conditions which they had found distressing or excessively uncomfortable, but which were not recorded as complications in the obstetric records. These included constipation (2), haemorrhoids (4), stress incontinence (1), urine retention requiring catheterisation (4) and painful stitches (6), as well as additional reports of anaemia (4), depression (3), raised blood pressure (2) and superficial phlebitis (1).

Both mothers and babies stayed in AMH significantly longer in 1951 than in 1985 (Table 8.11). The number of days in hospital has been calculated by subtracting the date of delivery from the date of discharge. Mothers of surviving singletons were in AMH on average 8.8 days in 1951 and 6.3 days in 1985; comparable figures for their babies were 9.5 and 6.6 days respectively. The mother's stay in hospital after a CS had been reduced from an average of 15.5 days in 1951 (range 12-20) to 9.3 days in 1985 (range 6-15).

While 46% of mothers in the recent sample had been discharged within five days only 3% of the 1951 sample had gone out by this time and this included hospital transfers. Conversely, few mothers in 1985 were detained for 10 or more days, 4% compared with 30% in 1951.

Because more babies were admitted to the Special Nursery for longer periods in 1951 more mothers went home leaving their babies in AMH—8% compared with 1% in 1985. In 1951 two mothers with their babies were

TABLE 8.11

LENGTH OF STAY IN HOSPITAL FOR MOTHERS AND BABIES—SURVIVING SINGLETONS ONLY

	1951		1985	
No. of days	No.	%	No.	%
Mother—5 and under	6†*	3	70	46
6–9	137†	67	76	50
10 or over	62	30	7	4
Baby—5 and under	6†°	3	70	46
6–9	128†	62	74	48
10 or over	71	35	9	6
No. of mothers and babies	205	100	153	100
Mean—mother	8.8 ± 2.88		6.3 ± 1.47	
		t = 9.82 p ⩽ 0.001		
baby	9.5 ± 2.85		6.6 ± 1.53	
		t = 11.43 p ⩽ 0.001		

* = One mother with active pulmonary TB transferred to City Hospital
† = One mother and baby discharged to City Hospital because of infection
° = One baby alone transferred to Children's Hospital for surgery

transferred to the City Hospital on account of infections, although both continued to breast feed; also one mother with active TB went there leaving her baby in the Nursery. Only one baby went out of AMH before the mother, being transferred to the Children's Hospital on the second day for surgery and being detained there for fourteen days; the mother was in AMH for six days and continued to supply breast milk. In 1985 there were no transfers of mothers to other hospitals and the only baby transferred for heart surgery, died.

The outcome of the first pregnancies of women in the two samples 34 years apart were remarkably similar, as were the birthweights of the babies. Infant feeding in AMH reflects the hospital policy which insisted on breast feeding in the early 1950s, but allowed a choice in the mid 1980s. Women in professional, technical and clerical occupations were more likely to breast feed, but the attitude expressed antenatally was important. There had been a change in the nature of problems arising in the puerperium—chest or urinary infections, genital sepsis and breast engorgement giving way to abdominal wound infections and iatrogenic problems. Both mothers and babies stayed in hospital significantly longer in 1951 and more mothers were discharged leaving their babies in the Special Nursery than in 1985, when overall fewer babies were admitted there.

## CHAPTER 9

Social Changes and the First Thirteen Postnatal Weeks

When their babies were thirteen weeks old the primiparae in both samples were visited at home, nearly always by the interviewer who had seen them antenatally. They were questioned about any changes in their housing conditions or social situation since the antenatal interview and about their experiences since leaving hospital.

All the postnatal data for 1985 were obtained at the home visit and the information is routinely available for 150 mothers who had 148 singletons and two pairs of twins. Four families had left Aberdeen, one couple, known to have separated, could not be traced, and the three women who had lost their babies, all of whom were still in contact with the obstetrician, were not visited.

The data for 1951 are more complicated as some items were introduced as the study progressed and not all the information was obtained at the 13 week postnatal visit. As described in Chapter 1, some questions, e.g. on contraception, were only asked of the random sample of mothers in the full social, dietary and psychological study who were still living in Aberdeen five years later, when they were invited to attend AMH to check on the child's health and development. Some families who had left Aberdeen (6) or were untraced (2) at 13 weeks were available to take part five years later (2). Five mothers had lost singleton babies and another had lost a twin. Therefore, in the analysis of the 1951 data the maximum, appropriate number of mothers or of singleton children varies from 128 to 200 according to the subject matter. Of the 200 mothers visited at home at 13 weeks, two had had twins.

Social Changes

HOUSING

Table 9.1 shows that the 1985 couples had been more mobile in that 19% had moved between the ANC interview and the 13 week postnatal visit compared with 11% in the earlier sample.

Most of the 1951 couples had moved from sharing a house either to other sublet accommodation or to rented homes (usually unfurnished) and

TABLE 9.1

HOUSING CHANGES AND CATEGORY

	1951 No.	1985 No.
Moved, category unchanged		
sub-let	10	—
rented unfurnished	—	4[4]
owner-occupier	—	11
Moved, category changed		
sub-let to rented furnished	1	—
sub-let to rented unfurnished	8	6 [6]
rented furnished to unfurnished	—	3 [2]
rented furnished to owner occupier	1	—
owner occupier to rented unfurnished	—	1 [1]
rented unfurnished to sub-let	2	1
Temporary accommodation	—	2
Total moved	22	28 [13]
not moved	178	122
% moved	11	19

( ) Council tenants

independent living arrangements. None had become council tenants. Trouble with an interfering landlady and with a neighbouring mother-in-law had driven two couples to give up their independent homes and to go and live with the husband's mother and the wife's parents respectively.

In contrast, 11 of the 28 couples in the current sample had sold their house and bought a new, usually larger one, and most of the remaining couples had been allocated a council house or been rehoused from substandard property. Two couples were in temporary accommodation at 13 weeks—one having sold their house prior to leaving Aberdeen, while the other was staying with the husband's parents while their own council house was being renovated. For medical reasons one couple had given up their own house and were staying with relatives.

HUSBAND'S OCCUPATION

Although 10% of husbands in the 1951 sample and 12% in the recent sample had changed their occupations and/or employers since the ANC interview, the overall occupational situation was unaffected.

Table 9.2 shows that in both samples men initially unemployed had found jobs whereas others had been paid off and some were unemployed at the 13 week postnatal visit. Men in both samples had changed jobs when they

TABLE 9.2

HUSBAND'S OCCUPATIONS—REASONS FOR CHANGES

Reasons for change	1951 No.	1985 No.
Unemployed—obtained job	1	2
Paid off—unemployed	2	1
new job	4	2
Completed training/apprenticeship	3	1
To avoid working away or unsociable hours	2	2
Better prospects	2	4
Demobbed/called up	4	—
Fear of redundancy	—	2
Other	3	4
Total changed	21	18
Total same job	179	132
% changed	11	12

completed training or an apprenticeship, or in order to avoid working away from home or unsocial hours, or for better prospects or for miscellaneous personal reasons. It was only in the early 1950s that men had been affected by demobilisation or a call-up to the Armed Forces. Fear of redundancy had influenced men in the recent sample to move to jobs which they thought would give them greater security.

WIFE'S RETURN TO WORK

By thirteen weeks postnatally, ten women in the 1951 sample (5%) and nine in the 1985 sample (6%) had returned to work. However, there were some important differences.

In 1951, all the ten mothers were doing manual, mainly unskilled work, all except two having returned to the job they had given up during pregnancy. Half the women worked full-time. Relatives, usually their mother with whom they lived, took charge of the baby.

In contrast, six of the nine mothers in the 1985 sample were in professional or clerical jobs; all except one was working for the same employer as antenatally. None were working full-time, most were doing part-time flexible or sessional work only. Seven of the women relied mainly on their husbands to look after the baby, but when necessary all were helped by other relatives or neighbours; one woman took the baby to a creche when she worked during the day.

Although most of the 1985 women who were in employment at thirteen weeks postnatally, had intended to return to work so soon after the birth, for others chance had intervened, e.g. request to help out an old employer in an emergency. It may be noted that a further fifteen of the 1985 mothers had made arrangements to return to their previous professional or technical jobs, eight of them full-time and seven part-time. In addition, one mother was actively looking for a secretarial job and another was planning to become a barmaid.

In the mid 1980s women who fulfilled a certain criteria, i.e. had been in a full-time job for at least two years (although some employers relaxed these criteria) could exercise an option antenatally which guaranteed their full-time job after maternity leave. Although the women were advised to keep their options open, of the 118 women in the 1985 sample who were eligible, only 63 had taken maternity leave and some of these had never intended to return to their job.

The First Thirteen Weeks

HELP ON DISCHARGE

The great majority of women, particularly in 1985, had received some help for a time after discharge from AMH. The marked changes in the source of help received (Table 9.3) reflect the changes in living conditions (Chapter 4) and the increased involvement of husbands.

In 1951, 39% of the mothers were already living with relatives, usually the wife's parents, nearly six times as many as in the 1985 sample. In contrast ten times as many, i.e. nearly half the mothers, in 1985 relied on their husbands although the majority had their mother and/or mother-in-law in Aberdeen available to help.

Sharing a home and having help readily available could be a mixed blessing as some husbands felt left out because there was 'nothing for them to do' with so many helpers on hand. However, there could be an advantage for the baby, e.g. one couple in 1951 were not really interested in their baby and were pleased to leave the grandparents to cope, while another couple

TABLE 9.3

HELP ON DISCHARGE

(n)	1951 (200)	1985 (150)
	%	%
Living with relatives	39	7
Husband only	5	49
Relatives came daily	13	15
Relatives stayed	6	8
Went to stay with relatives	12	4
Mixed help	2	7
Paid help	3	—
No help	20	10
Total	100	100

who resented having their sleep disturbed left the grandmother to deal with the baby during the night.

A similar proportion in each sample had relatives who came in regularly to help with domestic chores, but the help they gave varied from doing shopping or the daily washing (sometimes in the 1950s taking this away to do in their own homes with better facilities) to taking over all domestic responsibility. More mothers in the earlier sample went with their babies to stay with relatives for a while before returning to their own often cramped room(s) in old tenement property. Two of the six mothers in the recent sample who went to relatives when they left AMH did so because it was more convenient while their own homes were being modernised. However, all the women remained in Aberdeen, except for two in 1951 who went to relatives who lived in the country. Rather more 1985 mothers had relatives coming to stay with them, and more of these in 1985 came from outside Aberdeen (8 out of 12 compared with 5 out of 12 in 1951).

In 1951, one-fifth of the primiparae, twice as many as in 1985, maintained that they had had no help, but had managed on their own. This was not because relatives were not available, and only three such mothers in each sample did not have their own mother or mother-in-law in Aberdeen. They had wanted to establish their independence from the beginning, although many of them admitted that they had found it a great strain, as they had had little idea how much time had to be devoted to baby care and how tired they would become.

Six women in 1951 said that they had paid for domestic help—five women, four of whose husbands were in professional or managerial occupations, normally had daily help, and one woman had obtained a home help through the local authority service.

Women who had a home of their own had more choice about who would help them on their discharge from hospital and in which ways. In 1951 over half of such primiparae were helped by their own mothers, twice as many as in 1985. In contrast in 1985 nearly two-thirds of husbands were the main source of help and they usually took a week's holiday. Reliance on other relatives, and in particular on mothers-in-law had markedly declined (from 11% in 1951 to less than 2%). However, many were available in case of need.

HUSBAND'S HELP

The women were asked about the amount of help their husbands gave them in four aspects of baby care—bathing, changing nappies, bottle feeding and getting up in the night and whether they helped regularly, occasionally, or never.

Some husbands normally worked away from home, e.g. six in 1951 were serving overseas in the Armed Forces, whereas in 1985 husbands were more likely to be oilrig workers alternating two or three weeks off-shore with a similar period at home. All these husbands had spent some time at home since the baby was born and the assessment of their help relates to those periods.

Husbands in the 1950s took little part in baby care in the first 13 weeks—few in the earlier sample gave regular help and most had never bathed their babies, changed nappies or got up to attend to them in the night; also one-third had never given the bottle to babies receiving artificial or complementary feeding (Table 9.4). In the early 1950s many men, whatever their inclinations, were embarrassed about helping in the home or with the baby, which might make them out as 'a sissy'; however, receiving such help was often a source of pride to the wives. The idea was prevalent in some families that 'it was a terrible thing' for men to be involved in domestic chores or in baby care other than nursing. It was generally accepted that a man would not take a baby out on his own, though it would be acceptable to be seen helping his wife to push the pram up a hill.

Although most such restrictions were not evident in the mid 1980s, some ideas had not totally disappeared, and at least one 'modern' couple had difficulties with parents who held rigid views about the separate roles of men and women. Overall, husbands in the current study were more involved, not only when their wives and babies came out of hospital, but also on a regular basis. The mothers reported that more than half the 1985 husbands regularly gave the bottle if the infant was partly or entirely artificially fed (Table 9.4). A similar proportion regularly changed nappies, and more were willing to do so if disposable ones were being used or if they were wet rather than soiled. The husbands were less keen on bathing; the women described how the men felt that the babies were 'too small and delicate' for them to bathe, and fear of dropping 'a slippery handful' deterred them, although they might help with the preparations, and be delighted to play with the baby afterwards. Only 18% of husbands were said to regularly get up during the night if the baby needed attention although more were prepared to do so at weekends or when they were not working. However, nearly one-third had never been up during the night to attend to the baby. Most wives seemed happy with this arrangements, pointing out that it was unnecessary for both of them to be disturbed particularly if the baby was being breast fed—even so, a few husbands liked to be totally involved and would get up and bring the baby to bed for their wives to feed, and would change the baby

TABLE 9.4

HUSBANDS HELP WITH BABY—SINGLETONS ONLY

(n)	1951 (198)		1985 (148)	
	Regular	Never	Regular	Never
	% of sample		% of sample	
Bathing	4	68	38	33
Changing	1.5	58	57	7
Feeding*	2.5	33	58	4
Up at night	2	56	18	33

* Artificial or complementary feeding only

afterwards. By 13 weeks about 15% of babies were said to sleep through the night.

In both surveys there were some women who received no help from their husbands. In 1951 three couples were separated at the 13 week interview, including one where the husband denied paternity. (The only couple known to be separated in 1985 had to be excluded because the wife could not be traced.) A further three husbands were said to ignore their baby, one because the baby was not of the sex he had wanted. In the recent study, two husbands had warned their wives they were 'not baby persons', which the wives had not taken very seriously; although one had become 'a besotted dad', the other showed little interest, though his wife hoped that this would change as the child grew older. In addition, two wives reported that their husbands had been or were hostile to the baby. In one case the husband had lost his job about the time the baby was born which made him feel inadequate as a husband and father, but the couple were able to talk things through and matters improved once he got a new job. Another husband had reacted badly to his wife developing complications which led to a CS with subsequent problems and a prolonged stay in AMH—he was said to be angry about all this and to resent the baby because he felt neglected.

Occasionally, a husband would only tolerate a 'good baby' and at least two 1951 and one 1985 husbands were said to go out if the baby cried.

Mother at 13 Weeks

HEALTH OF MOTHER

At the 13 week postnatal interview all 1985 mothers and over 90% of those in 1951 were asked about their health since they had been discharged from AMH. More women had requested medical assistance in 1985, over one-half compared with one-third in 1951. The problems for which they had been treated or sought advice are listed in Table 9.5. Some women reported multiple problems. Not all contacts with their GP are included, as most women in both samples reported that the GP had called to see them and their babies as a matter of course when they got home; also consultations about contraception are not included.

In both studies some women had been in hospital and others had attended outpatient clinics, but no women reported both. In 1951 nine women—in addition to the three transferred direct from AMH, had been in hospital, two had suffered secondary PPH and had been readmitted for D and C, five had had breast abscesses excised while one of the remaining two had developed tuberculosis and the other an undiagnosed infection. In 1985 only three women had been in hospital, all readmitted for D and C on account of secondary PPH.

A further eight women in the 1951 sample and seven in the recent sample had attended outpatient clinics, and in both studies women had had breast abscesses excised and others had attended the dermatologist. Four women in

TABLE 9.5

HEALTH OF MOTHER IN 13 WEEKS AFTER DELIVERY

	1951 No. of women	1985 No. of women
Hospital in-patient		
Gynaecological—D & C	2	3
Breast abscess excised	5	—
Other—infections	2	—
Hospital out-patient		
Gynaecological/obstetric		
Perineal resutures	—	3
Pelvic X-ray	—	1
Other	4	—
Breast abscess excised	2	1
Skin clinic	2	1
Cardiology—ECG	—	1
GP consultations—some multiple complaints		
Breasts—abscess	10	—
mastitis	5	3
engorgement	2	1
Breast feeding problem	5	—
Lactation suppression	13	—
Vaginal—bleeding	2	8
infection/thrush	2	8
discharge	—	4
Wound/stitches infection—perineal	—	16
abdominal	—	1
Anaemia	1	5
Debility	7	—
Influenza/cold	4	7
Other	13	20
No. of women with problem(s)	61	78
No. of women with no problem	119	72
% with problem(s)	34	52

1951 had been seen at the gynaecological clinic on account of vaginal bleeding, ovarian cyst, retroverted uterus and vaginal discharge diagnosed as gonorrhea. Amongst the recent sample, three women had required resuturing of perineal wounds and two had required investigation—one had a pelvic X-ray following a CS, and the other who had been found to have a heart murmur, was sent for an electrocardiograph (ECG).

Only the GP had been consulted about the majority of health problems, but whereas in 1951 doctors had usually attended the women at home (89%) in 1985 most consultations had taken place in the surgery. The most common reasons for consulting the doctor were different for the two samples (Table 9.5). In 1951 problems were mainly about breasts and giving up breast feeding, whereas in 1985 vaginal bleeding and discharge as well as problems with perineal stitches and wound infections predominated.

Of those women who had stopped breast feeding since leaving AMH (102 in 1951 and 33 in 1985) a fairly similar proportion had encountered problems (14% and 15% respectively). While the 1951 women were more likely to have consulted their GP and been given stilboestrol in order to suppress lactation, in 1985 the women were more likely to have used cloth binders. Usually on the recommendation of their mothers some of the 1951 primiparae had obtained stilboestrol directly from the chemist or taken Epsom salts; one woman had used a vinegar and brown paper wrapper. Ten women in 1951 had consulted their GP about breast abscesses, but had not required hospital treatment.

The 1951 primiparae were more likely to report being 'run down' or debilitated whereas those in 1985 more often described themselves as 'anaemic'. A few women in each sample had had colds or influenza. Other conditions about which one or two women in each sample said they had consulted their GP were asthma, dermatitis, dizzy spells, eye problems, pyelitis and rashes. In 1951 GPs had also been consulted about boils, shingles and a second pregnancy, whereas in 1985 women had also attended their GPs on account of backache, haemorrhoids, and proteinuria.

Women did not always consult their GP about certain problems, e.g. a 1951 mother described how she had become very depressed and weepy for a time, and seven mothers in the recent sample were concerned about their difficulties in losing excess weight.

The preponderance of problems related to breasts and lactation in 1951 compared with 1985 reflects the change in hospital policy on infant feeding. Many 1951 primiparae went out of AMH with lactation well established, but unhappy about breast feeding and some never put the baby to the breast after discharge, either buying a bottle and a supply of dried milk on the way home or having made arrangements for them to be ready at home. Another change was that the 1951 practice of dosing with stilboestrol to suppress lactation was no longer favoured in 1985.

The prevalence of problems with wounds and stitches in 1985 was not found in 1951 when there was less obstetric intervention.

At 13 weeks one-tenth of women in each sample said that they had not made a complete recovery from the birth. Some of these women reported slow physical progress and generally feeling unwell; others complained of depression and excessive tiredness with feelings of being disorganised and unable to cope; a few said that they just did not enjoy motherhood and suffered accordingly. In the earlier sample marital problems, poor or difficult housing conditions and husbands being unemployed were also implicated. In 1985, of the four women who complained of depression, two gave family bereavement and one a housing problem as contributory factors in their lack of recovery and well-being. Also two women in 1985 said that they were still bleeding at 13 weeks. One had been switched from the progesterone only pill to the combined pill in an unsuccessful attempt to stop the bleeding and she was now waiting to be admitted for a D and C; the second woman had also been prescribed the pill to reduce the bleeding and was due for a further postnatal examination.

POSTNATAL EXAMINATION

Primiparae in the 1950s were more lax about attending for their postnatal check which in both periods was arranged for about six weeks after delivery. While only two women in the 1985 sample had failed to attend, one-quarter of women in the 1951 sample reported that they had not been. They variously said that they had forgotten about it, or lost their appointment card or did not think it was necessary because they were feeling well; a few who were attending their GP about the time of their appointment said they had been told not to bother. Three women were waiting for new appointments at 13 weeks, one being under pressure from her husband, who insisted on the need for a check-up.

All the postnatal examinations in the 1950s were at AMH whereas in the 1980s, although the majority of women attended the hospital, 43% of the recent sample had been to their GP under the arrangements for combined care (Hall *et al.*, 1980).

At their postnatal examination 17 women in each period were found to require treatment or further check-ups, representing 27% of the 1951 sample, but only 11% of the 1985 sample who attended. In each study there were women who were found to have inflammation, discharge, ovarian cyst, retroverted uterus, or to be still bleeding slightly or intermittently; in addition five women in the earlier study had pessaries fitted and one was to be readmitted as a stitch was causing abdominal pain and difficulty in micturition. There is some indication that the women in the 1950s were reluctant to consult their GP about vaginal inflammation and discharges and therefore those with problems were more likely to attend for their postnatal examinations.

CONTRACEPTION USED

As noted earlier, information on contraception is not directly comparable as it was obtained at different times and in different circumstances for the two samples. Data are only available for 125 of the 1951 sample and as they were giving their contraceptive history five years later (Thompson and Illsley, 1969) it was not possible to pinpoint actual use at 13 weeks, but only to identify the first contraceptive method to have been used after the first birth. In contrast, all the 1985 sample interviewed 13 weeks postnatally were asked about current use of contraception and about resumption of intercourse after the birth (see Appendix).

Table 9.6 gives details of postnatal contraception for those women in each sample for whom information is available.

Amongst the 1951 sample, considerably more used contraception after the birth than had done so before (72% and 45% respectively), and there had been an increase in mechanical methods, although none of the women fitted with a Dutch cap became regular users. In contrast there had been little change in the contraceptive practice of the 1985 couples although more women were favouring the IUCD, particularly at the expense of the diaphragm. Pill users who were breast feeding had switched to a progesterone only pill. One woman who had an elective CS had asked to be sterilised at the same time and this was considered advisable on grounds of age, obstetric problems and gynaecological condition. Three other women said that they had asked to be sterilised, but had been prescribed the pill for the time being.

In the 1950s doctors did not usually discuss contraception unless the woman raised the issue. However, the primigravidae who saw the psychologist in the course of the research had the opportunity to discuss the subject. Since from the mid 1960s the most efficient and favoured methods

TABLE 9.6

CONTRACEPTION AT 13 WEEKS POSTNATALLY

(n)	1951 (125) %	1985 (150) %
None	28	6
Coitus interruptus	25	1
Sheath	25	18
Safe period	1	1
Chemicals only	2	—
Diaphragm	15	1
Intra-uterine device	—	9
Pill	—	62
Mixed	4	1
Sterilised at Caesarean Section	—	1
Total	100	100

have been under medical control for many years contraception has been discussed individually as a matter of routine at AMH (Fullerton, 1973). By the time of the postnatal interview most primiparae in the recent survey had consulted a doctor about contraception—52% their GP, 20% AMH, and a further 7% had attended the Family Planning Clinic. However, over one-fifth of the sample said that they had not sought advice since the birth.

Most of the 1985 sample who had resumed intercourse without using contraception wanted another child quickly, as did one woman who had briefly used the pill. Others remained fatalistic, but said they 'would be quite happy' if they became pregnant.

Baby at 13 Weeks

FEEDING

Although more mothers in 1951 had left AMH breast feeding (90% compared with 60% in 1985) by 13 weeks the same proportion of babies in the two samples (38%) were getting some breast milk (Table 9.7). In 1985, however, rather fewer mothers were giving only breast milk and more were giving complementary artificial feeds. In addition, 70% of the 1985 mothers had started their babies on solid foods compared with only 2% in the 1951 sample (Table 9.8).

Amongst the mothers in the 1951 sample whose babies had left hospital on complementary feeds, nearly all had abandoned breast feeding by 13 weeks, compared with only half of the recent sample, all of whom were also giving their babies solid foods. One woman in each sample had phased out complementary feeds in favour of full breast feeding. Four women in the 1985 sample had continued a complementary feeding regime and three of them had also introduced solids.

Most babies in 1985 were taking solids by 13 weeks, but this was exceptional in 1951. Fully breast fed babies, however, were less likely to have been introduced to solids, 56% compared with 75% of artificially fed babies and 79% of those on complementary feeding regimes. Artificially fed babies tended to have solids introduced earlier and were the only ones who had been given solids before they were eight weeks old (Table 9.9). Whereas 57% of artificially fed babies had received solid foods by the time they were 10 weeks old, this applied to 25% of complementary fed babies and 21% of fully breast fed babies. This tendency for bottle fed babies to be started on solids early is not specific to Aberdeen, but was reported as a general phenomen by a Working Party on Child Nutrition (HMSO, 1980).

Mothers in all groups gave similar reasons for introducing solids—babies always seemed to be hungry, were never satisfied, would not settle, were fretful or had started to waken during the night. However, a few mothers

TABLE 9.7

DURATION OF BREAST FEEDING AT 13 WEEKS—SINGLETONS ONLY

	1951	1985
(n)	(198)	(148)
	%	%
Not started or abandoned in AMH	10	40
4 weeks or less	28	11
5–8 weeks	16	6
9–13 weeks	8	5
Still breast feeding	38	38
Total	100	100

TABLE 9.8

INFANT FEEDING ON DISCHARGE FROM AMH AND AT 13 WEEKS—
SINGLETONS ONLY

	1951				1985			
	On discharge from AMH				On discharge from AMH			
	Breast	Compl.	Artif.	Total	Breast	Compl.	Artif.	Total
(n)	(163)	(15)	(20)	(198)	(78)	(11)	(59)	(148)
At 13 weeks	%	%	%	%	%	%	%	%
Breast only	41	7	—	34	22	9	—	12
+solids	1	—	—	1	30	—	—	16
Complementary	4	—	—	3	3	9	—	2
+solids	—	—	—	—	10	27	—	8
Artificial only	54	86	100	61	6	—	30	16
+solids	—	7	—	1	29	55	70	46
Total	100	100	100	100	100	100	100	100

TABLE 9.9

WEEK SOLID FOODS INTRODUCED BY FEEDING AT 13 WEEKS—1985
SINGLETONS ONLY

	Breast	Complementary	Artificial
(n)	(23)	(12)	(69)
Week solids			
introduced	%	%	%
8 or less	—	—	19
9	13	17	16
10	8	8	22
11	22	33	9
12	35	42	27
13	22	—	7
Total	100	100	100
Mean weeks	11.4 ± 1.31	11.0 ± 1.17	10.0 ± 2.87

$$\lambda^2_{(10)} = 91.8 \quad p \leqslant 0.001$$

just felt that as time went on babies should begin to taste different foods. Although most mothers were aware that professional advice was not to give solids until babies were three to four months old, they were prepared to use their own discretion. Usually the babies were started on cereals, e.g. baby rice, softened rusks and fruit purees.

Many women who abandoned breast feeding did so after going home within the first rather than in the second or third month (Table 9.7). The relatively high proportion who gave up within a month in the earlier sample (28% compared with 11% in 1985) reflects the pressure in favour of breast feeding brought to bear on them in hospital, where they conformed sometimes against their inclinations, as discussed elsewhere. Most women, however, gave other reasons for stopping breast feeding (Table 9.10).

The main reason for abandoning breast feeding has been classified, taking full account of the mothers' statements and any circumstantial evidence. An inadequate supply of milk was the most usual reason given, although few babies had been test weighed and most had been doing well. The mothers usually inferred that they had insufficient milk because they said that the babies always seemed to be hungry and did not settle between feeds. However, particularly in 1951 there was often a strong element of the mothers being unhappy with breast feeding because they 'couldn't see how much the baby was getting', or they were embarrassed due to a lack of privacy in some shared homes. In both samples cracked and bleeding nipples had caused some women to stop breast feeding and in addition more women in the earlier sample blamed breast abscesses and mastitis.

Some mothers said that they had stopped breast feeding because they were unwell. Mothers in both periods mentioned having flu but usually they complained of something unspecific such as feeling 'very tired', or just 'unwell'. Also in 1951 bronchitis and having 'dizzy spells' were mentioned. A similar proportion of mothers in each of the samples said that they did not enjoy breast feeding and soon gave up. Plans to return to work led two mothers in the earlier sample and one in the recent to stop breast feeding. In 1951 three mothers said they had been persuaded by family members (2 mothers, 1 husband) that artificial feeding was better.

A few babies had had problems which caused the mothers to stop breast feeding. In the 1951 sample, five babies had been ill with pyloric stenosis, gastro-enteritis or vomiting, while two babies continued to have difficulties

TABLE 9.10

MAIN REASON BREAST FEEDING ABANDONED AFTER DISCHARGE FROM AMH

(n)	1951 (102) %	1985 (33) %
Inadequate lactation	45	43
Problems with breast and nipples	17	12
Maternal illness	10	15
Infant illness or difficulties	7	15
Mixed medical reasons	5	—
Disliked breast feeding	11	12
Returning to work	2	3
Influence of others	3	—
Total	100	100

in fixing. Similar problems with fixing and slow feeding made two mothers in the 1985 sample give up breast feeding. A further three who had been complementary feeding changed to full artificial feeding—two mothers explained that their babies seemed to prefer the bottle feeds, and the third who had expressed milk and given it by bottle because the baby had never taken to the breast, decided that artificial feeding would be easier.

HEALTH OF BABIES

Overall, more babies in 1985 had been seen at hospital or by the GP (72% compared with 59% in 1951). A similar proportion (8%) of babies in each sample had spent some part of their first 13 weeks in hospital, but twice as many in the present sample had been outpatients (9% compared with 4% in 1951). No baby had been both an inpatient and an outpatient. Table 9.11 lists the conditions as reported by the mothers for which infants had attended hospital or their GP.

Babies in both samples had been admitted to hospital on account of pyloric stenosis, congenital anomaly (oesophageal atresia in 1951 and Hirschsprung's disease in 1985), for chest infections and for observation for possible pancreatic abnormality. Vomiting, gastro-enteritis, ear, nose and throat infections and fractures of the thigh and of the skull accounted for the admission of the remaining 1951 infants. In contrast additional admissions in the recent sample were for hernia, poor weight gain, suspected fits, haematemesis, and checks as a precautionary measure on babies with heart murmurs.

More 1985 babies had attended outpatient clinics for checks on conditions noted in AMH, e.g. clicking hip, jaundice, hypospadias, heart murmur, a large head which was checked by a brain scan, and a lump in the neck. One infant developed a hernia, while two others had precautionary check-ups after one had been accidentally dropped and another had been found difficult to waken. In contrast only two 1951 babies were followed up as outpatients, one for assessment of general development and the other because the mother had been treated for syphilis. Other conditions for which babies in the earlier study had been referred to outpatient clinics were an injured shoulder, eczema, rashes, septic finger, and one infant received a course of heat treatment.

Some conditions had been treated only by the GP in both periods, predominantly colds and chest infections (Table 9.11) but also vomiting, colic, constipation and rashes. GPs had attended babies in the 1951 study for umbilical bleeding or infection, breast feeding difficulties, gastro-enteritis, inflamed vaccination scars, measles, swollen neck glands and poor weight gain. GPs had seen babies in the recent study on account of tongue tie, undescended testicles, sticky or inflamed eyes, thrush, eczema, ear infection and jaundice.

The GPs in 1951 had usually attended the babies at home (77%) whereas in 1985 most babies had been seen at the surgery (81%).

TABLE 9.11

HEALTH OF BABIES IN FIRST 13 WEEKS—SINGLETONS ONLY

	1951 *No. of babies*	1985 *No. of babies*
Hospital in-patient		
Treatment/observation for neonatal condition		
Pyloric stenosis	1	2
Congenital anomaly	1	1
Heart	—	2
Pneumonia/chest infection	4	2
Vomiting	4	—
Gastro-enteritis	2	—
Hernia	—	1
Fractures	2	—
Ear, nose and throat	2	—
Poor weight gain	—	2
Observation	1	2
Hospital out-patient		
Checks on neo-natal conditions		
Clicking hip	—	3
Jaundice	—	3
Hypospadias	—	1
Miscellaneous	2	3
Accidents	1	1
Skin	3	—
Hernia	—	1
Other	1	1
GP consultations		
Cord bleeding/infection	3	—
Congenital anomalies	—	3
Colds/chest infection	20	32
Breast feeding difficulties	18	—
Vomiting	1	3
Gastro-enteritis	1	—
Colic/fretful	6	15
Constipation	5	2
Rashes	2	16
Eye inflammation/stickiness	—	15
Thrush	—	9
Vaccination/septic	3	—
Other	4	2
No. of infants with problem(s)	117	107
No. of infants with no problem	81	41
% with problem(s)	59	72

MAIN PERSON CONSULTED

The primiparae in both samples were asked who was the first person they would turn to if they were worried or had a problem with the baby. Nearly half the women in 1951 named their mother as their first and main source of advice (Table 9.12). A further 6% mentioned other relatives, mainly sisters, but also mothers-in-law and aunts. In the recent sample, however, only one-fifth said it would be their mother (21%) and somewhat fewer than in 1951 named relatives (5%). In 1985, they were more likely to consult a health visitor, their husband or a friend.

In the early 1950s many primiparae seemed very passive and under the domination of their mothers who, if they did not actually live with them, often stayed nearby, and in some cases complained of and occasionally ridiculed 'all the fuss made about having babies', compared to what had happened in their own experience. In the recent study, primiparae frequently discussed how they and their parents recognised that things had changed and that the older generation were out of touch with developments. Thus, although many still consulted their mothers, more took professional advice or relied on their peers.

One couple in each sample had eventually broken off relations with an interfering relative—a maternal aunt and a mother-in-law respectively, in the latter case when the young mother involved said that she reached such a pitch that she 'was almost suicidal'. On the other hand, the arrival of the baby sometimes improved relationships, as in the case of one young mother and her formerly estranged mother-in-law.

Very few women said they would rely entirely on their own judgement in deciding what was necessary for their baby. One woman in the recent sample said she would consult the National Childbirth Trust, while another said she would consult books and literature. About one-tenth in each period said that they would go directly to their GP.

TABLE 9.12

MAIN PERSON CONSULTED ABOUT INFANT

(n)	1951 (182) %	1985 (150) %
General practitioner	11	10
Health visitor	28	35
Husband	3	17
Mother	48	21
Other relative	6	5
Friend	2	8
Self	2	3
Other	—	1
Total	100	100

Health visitors had played a much more active part in advising mothers in the mid 1980s than in the early 1950s when the service was very limited in the number of its staff and the scope of its work. An important aspect of the present service is a 24-hour telephone call system whereby a mother can get advice at any time. Indeed 48% of the primiparae said that they had phoned for assistance or advice even during the night. Many of the women, nearly all of whom had a telephone in their house, said that just knowing that the service was there in case of need had given them confidence. Most commonly the women had wanted advice about feeding, how to deal with a screaming or fretful baby, or with one who was being sick (Table 9.13). A call for help was usually followed quickly by a home visit. Often the problems were of a minor nature, but the health visitors had considered one-sixth of them sufficiently serious to refer the mother to the GP, particularly in cases of vomiting or colic.

TABLE 9.13

REASON MOTHER REQUESTED ADVICE FROM HEALTH VISITOR ABOUT THE BABY—1985 SAMPLE ONLY

Problem	No. of Infants
Feeding	17 [1]
Screaming/fretful	13 [2]
Vomiting	11 [3]
Colic	8 [3]
Rash	6
Constipation	4
Cold	3 [2]
Nose bleed	2
Other	8 [1]
Total infants with problems	72 [12]

(   ) Advised to consult GP

Health visitors at the time of both studies paid routine visits to mothers at home after the days of statutory care by midwives ended. Ten women in 1951 and two in 1985 maintained that a health visitor had never called on them. The information on the number of visits made was collected in rather different ways in the two studies, but the data indicate that the 1985 sample were visited more regularly. In each sample, however, 4–5% had received more than ten visits. Extra visits had usually been to monitor babies who had colic, who screamed incessantly, or had been of low birthweight or following a telephone request for advice.

In both studies, mothers were advised to attend a child welfare clinic, the staff of which usually included the local health visitor in order to maintain continuity with the families. Once again, the 1951 primiparae were more lax about taking their babies to these clinics—21% failed to attend, whereas in 1985 all mothers had been and they had attended more frequently (Table 9.14). In recent years, since the reorganisation of services, the mothers knew that a GP would be available to deal with any problems and that encouraged them to attend and to some extent served to increase GP consultations in 1985. However, most women in both periods emphasised that they went primarily to have the baby weighed. Some mothers in the earlier study preferred to have this done at the chemist's shop to avoid undressing the baby which was required at the clinic.

TABLE 9.14

ATTENDANCE AT CHILD WELFARE CLINICS

	1951	1985
(n)	(188)	(148)
Time attended	%	%
None	21	—
Occasionally or 1–3	18	9
Less than fortnightly or 4–6	27	51
At least fortnightly or regularly 7+	34	40
Total	100	100

CHAPTER 10

Some Associations with Occupations

In the 1950s research focused on the marked social class differences, based on the husband's occupation, in many of the characteristics studied. For example, women in the upper social classes were taller, older when they had their first baby, more educated, more likely to breast feed and to seek professional advice; for their part women in the lower social classes were more likely to be native Aberdonians, to have conceived before marriage and to have a low birthweight baby (Illsley, 1956a). The woman's own occupation was considered primarily in relation to work during pregnancy (Illsley et al., 1954). For present purposes, the occupations of both the husbands and wives have been used in the analysis in order to identify continuing associations and changing influences.

The husbands' occupations have been divided into three groups, namely: (1) non-manual, i.e. social classes I, II and III NM; (ii) skilled manual, i.e. social class III manual; and (iii) other manual, i.e. social classes IV and V. (GRO, 1950; OPCS, 1980). The women's occupations have been divided into three groups, namely (i) professional technical and clerical; (ii) distributive and skilled manual; and (iii) other manual. On account of the preponderance of clerical workers in the 1985 sample, the data have been reanalysed differentiating the professional and technical workers from those in clerical jobs.

Table 10.1 shows that some trends with occupation had persisted with only minor inconsistencies due to small numbers. In general, in both surveys, low occupational status was associated with an excess of wives and husbands who had been brought up in Aberdeen, who had a minimum of education, and who married during pregnancy; also in wives who saw their mothers more than weekly. In contrast, such occupations had the lowest percentage of couples living on their own and of wives being aged 25 or more at delivery.

Although the trends were still present in 1985, some overall social changes had had a marked effect, e.g. most couples in all groups had a home of their own (Chapter 4). Also, few women in the recent study had conceived prenuptially due to the revolution in contraceptive behaviour (Chapter 5).

In 1951 the only characteristic considered in Table 10.1 which showed a clearer trend with the wife's rather than the husband's occupation was her education—perhaps not surprisingly in view of the inter-relationship of education and occupation. However, in 1985 there were additional

TABLE 10.1

PERCENTAGE OF OCCUPATIONAL GROUPS WITH CERTAIN CHARACTERISTICS IN 1951 AND 1985 OCCUPATIONAL TRENDS PERSISTED

| | Wife's occupation | | | | | | | | | Husband's occupation | | | | | |
| | 1951 | | | 1985 | | | | | | 1951 | | | 1985 | | |
(n)	1 (63)	2 (88)	3 (62)	1 (113)	† (54)	2 (34)	(59)	3 (11)	(45)	1 (39)	2 (108)	3 (66)	1 (68)	2 (60)	3 (30)
Brought up in Aberdeen:															
Wife	58	82	75	50	†31	71	71	82	73	58	75	79	45	63	70
Husband	60	74	82	49	†37	68	49	51	59	51	76	79	38	68	63
Left school at minimum age															
Wife	50	97	98	31	†11	71	47	91	75	61	83	97	23	56	67
Husband	68	98	93	38	†28	68	47	91	73	58	93	96	21	60	87
Conceived prenuptially	19	31	38	7	†4	9	10	9	9	13	29	40	3	7	20
Wife sees mother more than weekly antenatally	61	75	75	48	†36	55	58	70	59	60	72	78	43	53	62
Unshared home	61	32	19	90	†90	91	90	80	88	68	35	21	95	90	78
Wife aged 25+ at delivery	45	34	27	68	†72	32	65	18	29	61	30	30	74	50	30

Wife's occupation:
1. Professional, technical and clerical
2. Distributive and skilled manual
3. Other manual

1† Professional and technical
2† Clerical
3† Other

Husband's occupation:
1. Non-manual
2. Skilled manual
3. Other manual

characteristics for which the wife's occupation, irrespective of which classification was used, was more discriminating, i.e. whether the couple had been brought up in Aberdeen, the frequency with which the wife saw her mother and the wife's age at delivery. Trends were more marked using the wife's occupation when professional or technical workers were differentiated from clerical workers. For example, whereas 11% of professional and technical workers had had a minimum of education, this applied to 49% of clerical workers; also whereas 36% of professional and technical workers saw their mothers more than weekly, 58% of clerical workers did likewise.

Using this redivision of occupations for wives in the 1985 sample, certain characteristics showed a clear trend not otherwise defined. Associated with increasing occupational status were cohabitation before marriage, the wife being aged twenty-three or more at marriage and the husband aged twenty-six or more, the wife working until at least 28 weeks gestation, and the husband being aged twenty-seven or more when he became a father (Table 10.2). Conversely, first meeting casually was a feature of declining occupational status.

Three characteristics showed a change in their association with occupation between the two samples (Table 10.3).

1. Height. In 1951 the percentage of tall women (5 ft 4 in and over) declined steadily with decreasing occupational status of either the husband or wife. In 1985, however, the lowest percentage of tall women was amongst clerical workers. Husbands in non-manual work had the highest proportion of tall wives, the lowest proportion was found amongst the wives of skilled manual workers. All occupational groups had experienced an increase in maternal height, but differential increases have narrowed the gap between them.

2. Contraceptive failure. In 1951 there was a marked social gradient in the reporting of contraceptive failure, the percentage being three to four times greater among the semi-skilled and unskilled manual worker husbands and wives respectively. As discussed in Chapter 5 the revolution in use of contraception and in the planning of pregnancy had meant that the few failures reported in 1985 were more random.

3. Frequency mother-in-law seen. In 1951 the proportion of women who saw their mother-in-law more than weekly increased with declining occupational status. This gradient was not found in 1985 when the highest proportion was amongst the wives of skilled manual workers or women who were either clerical workers or semi-skilled and unskilled manual workers.

In view of the high, but decreasing, proportion of women brought up in Aberdeen, the analysis was redone on this population only. The same patterns emerged as for the total sample except for the frequency with which the women saw their mothers and mothers-in-law. In each period there was relatively little difference for these characteristics between the occupational groups in this sedentes sample. In 1951, the proportion of women in the

TABLE 10.2

PERCENTAGE OF OCCUPATIONAL GROUPS WITH CERTAIN CHARACTERISTICS IN 1951 AND 1985
CONSISTENT TREND IN 1985 WHEN WIFE'S OCCUPATION RECODED

	Wife's occupation						*Husband's occupation*					
	1951			1985			1951			1985		
	1	2	3	1	2	3	1	2	3	1	2	3
(n)	(63)	(88)	(52)	(113)	(34)	(11)	(39)	(108)	(66)	(68)	(60)	(30)
				†(54)	(59)	(45)						
Couple met casually	25	29	19	34	50	36	14	31	22	25	48	47
				†30	37	47						
Couple cohabited				25	12	18				23	24	17
				†34	18	14						
Age at marriage:												
Wife 23 and over	49	43	37	44	27	36	74	37	35	39	47	27
				†50	39	29						
Husband 26 and over	48	31	32	35	24	45	64	31	32	32	32	33
				†41	29	29						
Wife stopped work 28 + weeks pregnant	26	15	25	71	38	45	26	19	25	75	53	51
				†77	64	40						
Husband at delivery aged 27 and over	55	36	38	61	38	54	77	35	35	72	43	40
				†69	54	42						

Wife's occupation:
1. Professional, technical and clerical — 1† Professional and technical
2. Distributive and skilled manual — 2† Clerical
3. Other manual — 3† Other

Husband's occupation:
1. Non-manual
2. Skilled manual
3. Other manual

TABLE 10.3

PERCENTAGE OF OCCUPATIONAL GROUPS WITH CERTAIN CHARACTERISTICS IN 1951 AND 1985
SOCIAL CLASS TREND MODIFIED

	Wife's occupation						Husband's occupation					
	1951			1985			1951			1985		
	1	2	3	1	2	3	1	2	3	1	2	3
(n)	(63)	(88)	(62)	(113) / †(54)	(34) / (59)	(11) / (45)	(39)	(108)	(66)	(68)	(60)	(30)
Maternal height 5 ft 4 in or over	38	22	10	43 / †48	47 / 37	45 / 47	44	23	11	55	35	40
Contraceptive failure	22	29	80	5	—	10	20	34	62	6	2	4
Mother-in-law seen more than weekly	44	50	56	22 / †18	18 / 26	36 / 24	36	51	52	19	30	23

Wife's occupation
1. Professional, technical and clerical
2. Distributive and skilled manual
3. Other manual

1† Professional and technical
2† Clerical
3† Other

Husband's occupation:
1. Non-manual
2. Skilled manual
3. Other manual

three occupational groups who saw their mother more than weekly varied between 82–90%; comparable figures for women seeing their mother-in-law were 54–62%. In 1985, taking the three groups as professional and technical/ clerical/ and the remainder, 78–86% of women in the groups saw their mother more than weekly and 30–34% saw their mother-in-law as frequently.

POSTNATAL SAMPLES

The postnatal factors were not so clearly related to the couples' occupations as were the characteristics discussed above. There was no association between either the woman's or her husband's occupation and her experience of analgesics or anaesthetics, of antenatal classes, the husband's help on discharge or with the baby. Numbers in some cases were of course small, e.g. those who had had a general anaesthetic. Other factors, e.g. husband's help, were to some extent affected by his conditions of work rather than the type of occupation *per se*. In some instances use of the wife's or husband's occupation tended to give conflicting results, e.g. whether the husband regularly bathed the baby.

Table 10.4 gives the factors related to the postnatal samples (singleton births only) where any occupational gradient was found using the wife's or husband's occupation in either or both studies. Although the wife's occupation tends to be more discriminating, the classification used can be important. For example in the 1985 study, the breast feeding history of clerical workers was very different from that of women in professional occupations, but fairly similar proportions in the two groups were giving the baby solids at 13 weeks.

Allowing for minor discrepancies due to small numbers, the proportion of LBW babies and of babies artificially fed at 13 weeks increased with decreasing occupational status in both samples. This also applied to artificial feeding on discharge from AMH in the recent study, but not in the earlier one when breast feeding in AMH was mandatory (see Chapter 8). This well known hospital policy undoubtedly inhibited many women from expressing a preference, but in 1985 when they had a choice, a definite intention to breast feed was directly associated with increasing occupational status.

Few babies in the 1951 sample had been given solids in the first three months. In the recent sample, analysis by the husband's and wife's occupation gave somewhat different results. The proportion of mothers who had given the baby solids increased with decreasing occupational status of husbands. The results are not so clear by the wife's occupation, as nearly all the distributive and skilled manual workers had given solids; the lowest proportion to have done so being in the semi-skilled and unskilled manual group and in clerical workers.

In general in both studies, the semi-skilled and unskilled manual worker or wives of men in similar low status occupations were least likely to seek help first from professionals if they had a problem with the baby, according to statements made during the postnatal interview (Table 10.4).

TABLE 10.4

PERCENTAGE OF OCCUPATIONAL GROUPS WITH CERTAIN CHARACTERISTICS IN 1951 AND 1985
POSTNATAL SAMPLES—SINGLETONS ONLY

	Wife's occupation						Husband's occupation					
	1951			1985			1951			1985		
	1	2	3	1	2	3	1	2	3	1	2	3
(n)	(56)	(83)	(59)	(107) †(49)	(31) (58)	(10) (41)	(37)	(104)	(57)	(63)	(59)	(26)
Low birthweight baby	2	10	10	5 †4	13 5	10 12	—	9	11	5	7	12
Positive intention to Breast Feed	59	56	51	65 †82	51 52	22 45	56	57	52	71	58	33
Baby fully breast fed on discharge from AMH	86	78	81	58 †73	42 45	30 39	84	81	81	63	46	42
at 13 weeks	59	29	22	35 †53	29 21	20 27	49	37	26	52	17	23
Solids introduced by 13 weeks	3	2	7	68 †71	90 65	60 83	8	3	2	63	78	81
Wife would consult GP or HV first with baby's problems	14	10	10	45 †45	39 45	30 37	12	15	4	41	44	42

Wife's occupation:
1. Professional, technical and clerical
2. Distributive and skilled manual
3. Other manual

1† Professional and technical
2† Clerical
3† Other

Husband's occupation:
1. Non-manual
2. Skilled manual
3. Other manual

In view of the importance of cultural and familial influences in childcare, and the different composition of the two samples, the data were reanalysed for women brought up in Aberdeen. The percentage and patterns in the 1951 study were little changed from those of the total sample. In the recent study, however, trends persisted but were more marked. For example, the percentages of women fully breast feeding on discharge from AMH were 69, 37 and 27 for the groups of professional and technical, clerical and other workers respectively. The larger population of in-migrants in the 1985 sample (Chapter 3) undoutedly served to modify the overall figures, particularly in favour of breast feeding and consulting professionals in all groups. On the other hand, in-migrants in professional, technical and clerical occupations were more likely to have had a LBW baby and to have introduced solids to baby feeding by 13 weeks, compared with sedentes in similar occupations.

More detailed analysis is not feasible because of small numbers and the complex variations in attitudes and behaviour.

## CHAPTER 11

The Weighed Diet Surveys

The method adopted for the 1951 survey after preliminary experiments, the mode of analysis and the results have been reported by Thomson (1958, 1959*a*, *b*). Both the 1951 and the 1985 surveys were based on the weighing of food for one week in the seventh month of pregnancy using spring balances. The dietitian visited the women two or three times in the course of the 1951 survey, whereas in 1985 the women were seen only at the Antenatal Clinic, although the dietitian was always available by phone to deal with queries. Both the surveys were based on random samples of primigravidae booked for hospital confinement, and for present purposes only those records which in 1951 overlapped with the social enquiry and were in the random sample have been used, which means that to some extent upper social class primigravidae are under-represented (Chapters 1 and 2).

RATIONING AND WELFARE FOODS

Rationing was still in force in 1951 and the levels of adult entitlement per week are given in Table 11.1 (Ministry of Food, 1954), but pregnant women could from time to time receive extra meat and eggs. In addition, under the Welfare Foods Service, expectant women were entitled to supplements available at clinics and various welfare centres (Ministry of Food, 1950).

TABLE 11.1

AVERAGE WEEKLY RATIONS—ADULT ENTITLEMENT 1950 and 1951

		1950	1951
Fresh carcase meat old pence		24.5	17.5
Bacon	oz	4.4	3.9
Butter	oz	4.4	3.7
Margarine	oz	4.0	4.0
Cooking fat	oz	2.1	2.0
Cheese	oz	2.0	2.0
Sugar	oz	10.6	11.8
Tea	oz	2.3	2.0

Taken from Ministry of Food, Domestic Food Consumption and Expenditure 1952; Annual Report of the National Food Survey Committee HMSO, 1954.

(a) 1 pint of milk daily for $1\frac{1}{2}$ old pence, as against the normal retail price of 5 old pence

(b) concentrated orange juice—a 6oz bottle for 5 old pence. The recommended daily dose provided 30mg of vitamin C and the bottle lasted 9 days

(c) cod liver oil—a 6oz bottle, or 45 chocolate coated vitamin A and D tablets free per six weeks. The normal daily dose of one teaspoonful of cod liver oil or one tablet provided a maximum of 4000 i.u. of vitamin A and 800 i.u. of vitamin D.

Both (a) and (b) were free to those who could not afford to pay. However, the full diet survey conducted between 1948–53 found a marked social class gradient in the uptake and use of all these welfare foods (Marr *et al.*, 1955). The dietitians reported a good deal of ignorance and apathy about such supplements, e.g. the vitamin tablets were thought to be laxatives. Although practically all primigravidae purchased the subsidised pint of milk it was seldom kept exclusively for their own use, e.g. from the weighed surveys, only 58% of SC I and II women took one pint of milk or more daily, and in SC IV and V only 18%. Even less use was made daily of the orange juice and vitamin concentrates.

CALCULATION OF NUTRITIVE VALUES

Thomson (1958) describes the method by which nutritive values were calculated for the 1951 diets. A composite table of values was derived from various sources including McCance and Widdowson (1946), the Medical Research Council: Accessory Food Factors Committee's (1945) 'Nutritive Value of Wartime Foods' and unpublished tables provided by the Chief Scientific Adviser (Food) to the Ministry of Agriculture, Fisheries and Food. This latter was used exclusively for the calculation of values of riboflavin and nicotinic acid. The energy values derived from the protein, fat and carbohydrate (CHO) content of each diet were calculated with the factors 4,9, and 3.75 Kcal/g respectively. Carbohydrate values expressed as starch in certain tables were brought into line with those of McCance and Widdowson, expressed as glucose, by multiplying by 1.12.

The recipes for cooked dishes used in the preparation of tables by McCance and Widdowson did not replicate those customarily used in Aberdeen. Therefore, all initial analysis was based on the nutritive values of 'edible portions of food as purchased'. Subsequently values for ascorbic acid and for thiamin were corrected for cooking losses according to the procedure recommended by the MRC: Accessory Food Factors Committee (1945). Thence, the total supply of thiamin was reduced by 15%, ascorbic acid from cooked green vegetables by 75% and from other cooked vegetables by 50%. Thomson (1958*a*) considered that this crude method of correction might result in considerable errors in the nutrient values. All the work in 1951 was done manually using desk calculators.

The situation was very different in 1985 since the development of

TABLE 11.2

COMPARISON OF NUTRITIONAL VALUES FOR TWO 1951 DIETS USING 1950 AND 1985 METHODS OF CALCULATION

| | | Diet 1 | | | Diet 2 | | | Diets 1 & 2 | | |
| | | Method | | | Method | | | Method | | |
		1951	1985	% difference	1951	1985	% difference	1951	1985	% difference
Energy	MJ	9.88	9.79	−1	9.59	10.24	+7	9.74	10.02	+2.8
Protein	g	74.00	81.50	+10	71.40	81.30	+14	72.70	81.40	+12.0
Fat	g	125.10	125.30	+1	86.80	99.30	+14	105.95	112.80	+6.5
Carbohydrate	g	249.50	233.30	−7	324.20	319.80	−2	286.85	276.50	−3.6

nutritional science had resulted in standards of nutritional values being produced and it was possible to use a computerised tape (Lowell and Mackie, 1983) obtained from the School of Nutritional Science at Robert Gordon's Institute of Technology in Aberdeen. The computer programme which calculated nutritional components for all foods was based on McCance and Widdowson's The Composition of Foods (Paul and Southgate, 1978). The weekly intake of each woman was converted into nutritional components and the computed results were used for analysis.

Recomputation of the 1951 diets in this way was not possible as the original records had been destroyed. Thus, direct comparison of the results for the two samples cannot be made, and only overall findings of associations of nutritional values with other variables can be presented. However, two complete records of menus and results were available from (non-pregnant) staff at the time (a dietitian and BT). These have been reprocessed, along with the 1985 diets.

It may be noted that energy in the recent survey was measured in Megajoules (MJ) and the Kilocalories (Kcal) used in the earlier survey were converted for comparison (1,000 Kcal = 4.2 MJ).

Table 11.2 shows the two 1951 diets with values recalculated in the same way as in the recent survey. Although some of the values are very similar, e.g. energy and fat of diet 1, intake of protein is 19-14% higher and of carbohydrate 6-2% lower in the two diets respectively. Recalculated values of calcium and some vitamins were only available for diet 1 and were all higher—calcium 4%, vitamin C 6%, nicotinic acid 8% and riboflavin 12%. These results tend to suggest that the method used to calculate the 1951 dietary intakes may give underestimates except for carbohydrate compared with that used in 1985, but whether this would be confirmed with bigger numbers is unknown. It must be stressed that for present purposes direct comparisons between group means must be interpreted with great caution due to differences in methodological factors including type of analysis.

However, the recent survey indicated a 20% reduction in energy intake by these Aberdeen primigravidae which is similar to the difference recorded between the National Food Survey for 1952 (MOF, 1954) and for 1984 (MOAFF, 1986) which was 19% less for a household of two adults only and 16% less for all households.

Changes with Time

Although the 1951 primigravidae were still subjected to some rationing of staple foods and had experienced all the propaganda of the wartime Ministry of Food, diet was not of any great concern to them. Some women had no responsibilities for meals as many still lived in a parental home as described in Chapter 4. The dieticians (Hope et al., 1956) reported:

> In general we found that food and cooking were topics of very limited interest to most of these women. Their habits were conservative and seemed to be little

influenced, if at all, by experience of school meals, works canteens, and by food education generally. Though many knew quite well 'what was good for them' relatively few applied their knowledge in defiance of long-established custom. Unless they had been accustomed, as children and adolescents, to a good varied diet, they simply continued to take, after marriage, the stereotyped but easily prepared meals that their mothers had cooked before them. The composition of many of the meals shows that, in Classes III, IV and V at least, to eat according to the patterns advocated by some nutritional authorities would involve a very considerable change of custom. . . . Conservative attitudes, together with ignorance, are undoubtedly at the root of some of the unsatisfactory habits we observed.

In marked contrast, the dietitian in the recent study found that the majority of the primigravidae were interested in nutrition and a few were very concerned about taking 'a good diet'. In addition to this interest, co-operation was facilitated by the fact that the vast majority of the primigravidae had their own well-equipped kitchen. Overall they tended to be aware of the importance of good nutrition during pregnancy, and welcomed the opportunity to take part in a diet-related research project.

About half the 1985 women wanted detailed comments on their diet when they reviewed the week's record with the dietitian and about one-quarter specifically asked how to improve their diet. Interest was shown in the effect of nutrition on the outcome of pregnancy and on infant feeding, and the primigravidae were also concerned about how they could regulate their diet postnatally in order to regain their pre-pregnancy weight.

A particular feature of the increased awareness of the importance of diet to health was that some women knew of the value of dietary fibre in avoiding or relieving constipation during pregnancy. Some women also considered that a weekly serving of liver was 'good for you', and this resulted in the high upper limit of vitamin A intake recorded in the 1985 study.

In the years between the two surveys, considerable changes had taken place not only in attitudes to diet and nutrition, but in the availability of foodstuffs and in social patterns relating to 'eating out'. In the early 1950s it was uncommon for pregnant women to go out for meals in restaurants, due in part to some reluctance to appear in public. This was no longer the case in the 1980s, and in addition there had been a great increase in the number of restaurants and other eating places open in the city. Many of the primigravidae were in the habit of eating out quite regularly.

Thirty women (21% of the 1985 diet sample) had a total of 20 lunches, 23 dinners and one breakfast out in the week in which they did the diet survey (approximately 1.4% of meals).

Lunches eaten out tended to be bar type or snacks, but there was much greater variety in evening meals eaten out which were usually taken in restaurants or hotels. Exceptionally, meals and in one case a mid-morning snack were taken in the homes of friends, not relatives. The women recorded details of any food eaten out and some from their experience of doing the survey or of cooking gave approximate quantities; however, after detailed discussion, the dietitian estimated quantities which were used in the analysis.

Whether eating out or at home, the primigravidae in the recent sample had ready access to a much bigger variety of foodstuffs than their counterparts in 1951. A whole range of goods not on sale in Aberdeen in the early 1950s were readily available in supermarkets and specialist food shops in the 1980s. Some foods almost, if not totally, unknown in Aberdeen in the early 1950s which featured quite frequently in the diets of the 1985 sample of primigravidae were for example, yoghurt (74), hamburgers (41), pizza (26) and lasagne (16); curry was also eaten by 21 women.

The variety of foods eaten by the primigravidae in the course of the survey had doubled from an average of 25.0 in 1951 to 49.9 in 1985. To some extent, however, this score is exaggerated. In the recent survey if in the course of a week the woman had taken a food cooked in different ways or with different ingredients added, each would have been counted in the variety score, but this did not apply in the earlier survey. The items most affected were likely to have been potatoes and cereals—potatoes may have been counted as 'one' in 1951 irrespective of how they were cooked, whereas chips, baked, boiled, or roasted potatoes would all have been counted separately in 1985. As the surveys applied to one week only this was unlikely to substantially affect the overall pattern.

There is no record of any alcohol being drunk in the 1951 survey, but 32 of the 1985 primigravidae had drunk some alcohol, but none regularly, during the survey week. Twenty-two women had drunk only white wine, but others had recorded red wine, advocat, bacardi, beer, sherry and vermouth, or a combination. Overall, however, the contribution of alcohol to energy was very slight.

Results

In considering the diets of the two samples only the diets which the dietitian accepted as reliable after checking with the women on details of items and weights recorded have been analysed. Diets were deemed unreliable if many items were not recorded or most weights were either missing or absurd or the record was so badly kept that it was worthless.

RELIABLE DIETS

More of the 1985 primigravidae provided a complete or reliable diet survey—92% compared with 80% in 1951. This reflects not only their greater interest in food and quantities and their greater familiarity with weighing and measuring, but also the fact that individual co-operation was facilitated by improved and independent living conditions. The few 1985 women whose dietary records were deemed unreliable showed no social class association in marked contrast to 1951 when significantly more were manual workers (Table 11.3). Similarly, their husbands were more likely to be in semi-skilled or unskilled manual occupations.

TABLE 11.3

RELIABILITY OF DIET SURVEY AND OCCUPATION

(n = 100%)	1951		1985	
	Reliable (94)	Unreliable (24)	Reliable (142)	Unreliable (11)
Wife's occupation	%	%	%	%
Professional and clerical	37	8	74	45
Distributive and skilled manual	41	38	20	46
Other manual	22	54	6	9
	$\lambda^2_{(2)}=11.85$ p$\leqslant$0.01		$\lambda^2_{(2)}=2.8$ N.S.	
Husband's occupation				
Non-manual	18	4	41	55
Skilled manual	56	33	41	18
Other manual	26	63	18	27
	$\lambda^2_{(2)}=10.84$ p$\leqslant$0.01		$\lambda^2_{(2)}=1.94$ N.S.	

The weeks of gestation in which the diet surveys were carried out were more concentrated in 1985 than in 1951 due to the design of the study and the relatively limited commitment of the dietitian. However, the vast majority of diet surveys in both periods refer to 29-32 completed weeks of gestation—77% in 1951 and 89% in 1985.

FOOD AND ENERGY AND SOME NUTRIENTS

Table 11.4 gives the means and range of items analysed in the two surveys. For every item there is a considerable range of values. Taken at their face value, but with the proviso stated earlier, the mean values in 1985 were significantly lower for energy, protein, fat, carbohydrate, thiamin and retinol equivalent, higher for nicotinic acid, but similar for the remaining items. A significantly higher proportion of energy was derived from protein in the 1985 diets while a significantly smaller proportion was accounted for by carbohydrate. However, the percentage of energy obtained from fat was similar (38%) in the two surveys. Table 11.5 shows the correlation coefficient between dietary components and with a few exceptions, e.g. ascorbic acid in 1985, they are all statistically significant, mostly at the 0.001 level, in both samples. This shows that overall diets high in one nutrient were likely to be high in others. It may be noted that, with few exceptions affecting carbohydrate, coefficients in 1951 were higher than in 1985.

SOME ASSOCIATIONS

In both 1951 and 1985, a positive association was found between dietary intake and the woman's height (Table 11.6). Thus, shorter women tended to eat less and particularly in 1951, to have a less varied diet. Highly significant associations were noted between height and energy, protein and carbohydrate intake for both surveys, but especially in 1985, and for fat only in the recent survey. The association between height and vitamin and mineral intake is less clear cut, with the only noteworthy association with height being found for calcium and riboflavin in 1985, while in 1951 strong associations were found with ascorbic acid and nicotinic acid and to a lesser extent, with thiamin. The proportion of energy obtained from protein, fat and carbohydrate did not vary with height group (Table 11.6).

For the purpose of statistical analysis, the influence of social class on height has been considered using a dichotomous division of occupations. The husband's occupation at the time the wife first attended the ANC has been divided between non-manual and manual and with the wife's main occupation before marriage divided between professional/technical/clerical and other occupations. For 1985, further analysis dividing the wife's occupation between professional/technical and other was done. Table 11.7 shows that when controlling for social class, irrespective of which occupational classification is used, the associations noted with height remain, although there are some minor differences in the degree of significance. Significant partial correlation coefficients were found between

TABLE 11.4

NUTRITIONAL VALUES—DAILY ENERGY COMPOSITION AND VARIETY SCORE: RELIABLE DIETS ONLY

		1951			1985			t test
		Mean	SD	Range	Mean	SD	Range	p≤1
Energy	MJ*	10.52	2.26	6.0–16.2	8.15	1.62	4.2–12.1	0.001
Protein	g	77.31	16.40	43.5–131.4	70.30	14.86	37.9–139.8	0.001
Fat	g	110.23	28.66	58.7–197.1	84.80	19.51	46.6–136.6	0.001
Carbohydrate	g	315.99	78.08	174.0–510.2	235.64	54.79	91.2–367.8	0.001
Calcium	mg	1068.34	336.97	306.0–1894.0	980.09	463.34	398.0–5238.0	NS
Retinol equivalent	µg	2404.50	745.66	150.6–2999.7	1318.10	1402.84	198.3–7153.36	0.001
Thiamin	mg	1.44	0.31	0.61–2.13	1.26	0.56	0.43–6.19	0.006
Riboflavin	mg	1.91	0.51	0.85–3.14	1.90	0.68	0.76–4.63	NS
Ascorbic acid	mg	94.50	38.72	21.0–207.0	86.23	72.20	11.0–644.0	NS
Nicotinic acid	mg	11.90	2.90	5.9–21.5	17.14	5.85	6.8–51.3	0.001
Variety score		25.04	6.01	13.0–47.0	49.90	10.93	22.0–80.0	0.001
% energy: Protein		12.60	1.60	9.2–18.9	14.80	2.25	10.5–21.1	0.001
Fat		38.60	3.81	26.3–48.0	38.50	4.40	26.5–49.6	NS
Carbohydrate		48.30	6.45	31.8–63.8	46.10	5.04	30.5–57.0	0.004

* 4.2 MJ = 1,000 Kcals

TABLE 11.5

CORRELATION COEFFICIENTS OF DAILY DIETARY INTAKE: * 1951—ABOVE †1985—BELOW

	Energy	Protein	Fat	CHO	Calcium	Thiamin	Riboflavin	Ascorbic acid	Nicotinic acid
Protein	0.84* 0.74†								
Fat	0.91 0.86	0.84 0.63							
Carbohydrate	0.70 0.87	0.41 0.52	0.45 0.58						
Calcium	0.61 0.34	0.71 0.38	0.57 0.26	0.37 0.27					
Thiamin	0.77 0.32	0.98 0.27	0.76 0.22	0.48 0.37	0.46 0.18				
Riboflavin	0.71 0.46	0.86 0.63	0.71 0.29	0.36 0.41	0.87 0.46	0.67 0.47			
Ascorbic acid	0.33 0.25	0.38 0.17	0.24 0.08	0.26 0.33	0.43 0.03	0.34 0.19	0.44 0.09		
Nicotinic acid	0.63 0.43	0.71 0.57	0.61 0.23	0.34 0.44	0.25 0.19	0.63 0.54	0.54 0.72	0.36 0.18	
Retinol equivalent	0.34 0.18	0.37 0.27	0.37 0.14	0.20 0.13	0.43 0.14	0.37 0.02	0.44 0.49	0.43 0.02	0.33 0.24

TABLE 11.6

MEAN DAILY NUTRIENT INTAKE, ENERGY CONSUMPTION AND VARIETY SCORE BY HEIGHT

(n)		1951				1985			
		Under 5ft 1in (14)	5ft 1in to 5ft 4in (55)	5ft 4in & over (25)	r‡	Under 5ft 1in (16)	5ft 1in to 5ft 4in (65)	5ft 4in & over (61)	r‡
Energy	MJ	10.1	10.2	11.5	0.25***	7.0	8.0	8.6	0.30****
Protein	g	73.0	75.2	84.3	0.22**	60.6	68.3	75.0	0.33*****
Fat	g	105.0	106.5	121.3	0.15	71.7	84.4	88.6	0.23*****
Carbohydrate	g	302.1	311.0	334.7	0.27***	203.9	234.1	245.6	0.25*****
Calcium	mg	1026.0	1042.5	1148.9	0.09	776.4	912.9	1105.1	0.25****
Retinol equivalent	µg	2273.2	2408.5	2486.2	0.11	1473.1	1001.7	1225.9	0.12
Thiamin	mg	1.4	1.4	1.5	0.20**	1.1	1.2	1.3	0.13
Riboflavin	mg	1.8	1.9	2.1	0.11	1.6	1.8	2.0	0.19**
Ascorbic acid	mg	80.8	88.2	116.1	0.34****	104.7	79.0	89.0	-0.03
Nicotinic acid	mg	11.2	11.5	13.3	0.27***	15.5	17.2	17.5	0.11
Variety score		22.2	23.9	28.7	0.41****	47.4	48.9	51.6	0.11
% energy: Protein		12.5	12.7	12.4		14.9	14.5	15.0	
Fat		38.4	38.7	38.9		37.9	38.8	38.3	
CHO		48.0	48.7	47.2		45.8	46.4	46.0	

‡ correlation coefficient of nutrient intake and variety score with height

**p ≤ 0.05
***p ≤ 0.01
****p ≤ 0.001

TABLE 11.7

PARTIAL CORRELATION COEFFICIENT OF DIETARY INTAKE WITH HEIGHT CONTROLLING FOR OCCUPATION

	1951 Partial correlation		1985 Partial correlation		
	Husband's occupation‡	Wife's occupation A	Husband's occupation‡	Wife's occupation A	B
Energy	0.25***	0.23***	0.30****	0.30****	0.30****
Protein	0.22**	0.20**	0.32****	0.35****	0.32****
Fat	0.15	0.13	0.23***	0.24***	0.24***
Carbohydrate	0.29***	0.27***	0.26****	0.25****	0.25****
Calcium	0.09	0.05	0.24***	0.27****	0.23***
Retinol equivalent	0.12	0.11	0.11	0.12	0.10
Thiamin	0.21**	0.22**	0.12	0.14	0.12
Riboflavin	0.11	0.07	0.19**	0.20***	0.17**
Ascorbic acid	0.33****	0.31***	−0.05	−0.02	−0.06
Nicotinic acid	0.27***	0.26***	0.12	0.13	0.10

Dichotomous division of occupations:
‡ Non manual/manual
A Professional, technical and clerical/other
B Professional and technical/other
   ** $p \leqslant 0.05$
  *** $p \leqslant 0.01$
 ****$p \leqslant 0.001$

height and energy, protein and carbohydrate intake for both surveys, although once again a significant association with fat intake only featured in 1985. These findings indicate that the noted association between height and dietary intake is not attributable to variations in the occupation of either partner.

The separate influences of the occupations of the woman and her husband on dietary intake are considered in Tables 11.8 and 11.9 respectively.

In 1951 wives with semi-skilled and unskilled manual jobs tended on average to eat less in energy, protein and fat than wives in professional and clerical occupations, whereas carbohydrate intake was slightly increased (Table 11.8). Wives in distributive or skilled manual occupations, however, ate least of all. The percentage of energy made up of protein, fat and carbohydrate was very similar between the occupational groups. Similarly, wives of husbands in semi-skilled and unskilled occupations ate less in energy, protein and fat than those in other occupational groups (Table 11.9). However, those with husbands in skilled manual jobs tended on average to eat similar amounts in energy, protein and fat as those whose husbands were in non-manual occupations, but they ate the most carbohydrate of all.

TABLE 11.8

MEAN DAILY NUTRIENT INTAKE, ENERGY COMPOSITION AND VARIETY SCORE BY WIFE'S OCCUPATION

(n)		1951 A (35)	1951 B (38)	1951 C (21)	1951 r‡	1985 A (105)(51) †	1985 B (28)(54)	1985 C (9)(37)	1985 r‡
Energy	MJ	11.0	9.9	10.6	-0.13	8.2 / 8.3	8.1 / 8.3	7.2 / 7.9	-0.11 / -0.06
Protein	g	80.9	73.0	78.0	-0.16	† 72.3 / 73.3	66.9 / 71.5	57.7 / 65.2	-0.22*** / -0.17**
Fat	g	115.6	104.5	109.2	-0.13	85.8 / 85.7	83.7 / 85.1	76.3 / 82.5	-0.10 / -0.02
CHO	g	321.7	303.9	325.2	-0.02	† 236.4 / 236.7	241.5 / 237.9	208.1 / 235.0	-0.03 / -0.02
Calcium	mg	1193.4	941.7	1053.3	-0.26**	1036.2 / 1126.4	846.6 / 955.0	740.9 / 826.7	-0.19** / -0.24****
Retinol equivalent	µg	2576.3	2322.3	2246.5	-0.18**	1384.5 / †1684.4	1343.7 / 1002.1	463.9 / 1154.3	-0.07 / -0.21***
Thiamin	mg	1.4	1.4	1.5	0.0001	1.3 / 1.3	1.1 / 1.4	1.0 / 1.1	-0.19** / -0.05
Riboflavin	mg	2.1	1.7	1.9	-0.24**	† 2.0 / 2.1	1.7 / 1.9	1.4 / 1.6	-0.20*** / -0.26*****
Ascorbic acid	mg	106.5	85.0	89.7	-0.24**	95.6 / 104.6	57.0 / 87.1	68.1 / 61.1	-0.20**** / -0.20****
Nicotinic acid	mg	12.2	11.6	11.9	-0.05	17.9 / †18.2	15.3 / 17.2	14.1 / 15.1	-0.19** / -0.20***
Variety score		29.1	23.5	21.0	-0.53****	51.3 / †51.9	48.7 / 50.8	37.7 / 45.9	-0.30**** / -0.16**

% energy									
Protein	12.6	12.6	12.7	†	15.0	15.2	14.2	14.8	13.6	14.1
Fat	38.8	38.9	37.9	†	38.5	38.2	38.4	38.9	39.4	38.7
CHO	47.5	48.7	48.8	†	45.7	45.7	47.2	45.7	46.5	47.0

** p < 0.05
*** p < 0.01
**** p < 0.001

Wife's occupation: A = professional, technical and clerical
B = distributive and skilled manual
C = other manual

A† = professional and technical
B† = clerical
C† = other

† Wife's occupation is a dichotomous variable divided between A/B + C or A†/B† + C† correlated with daily nutrient intake and variety score

TABLE 11.9

MEAN DAILY NUTRIENT INTAKE, ENERGY COMPOSITION AND VARIETY SCORE BY HUSBAND'S OCCUPATION

		1951				1985			
(n)		Non manual (17)	Skilled manual (53)	Other manual (24)	r‡	Non manual (58)	Skilled manual (58)	Other manual (26)	r‡
Energy	MJ	10.6	10.6	10.2	−0.007	8.2	8.1	8.4	−0.02
Protein	g	77.8	78.0	74.3	0.002	73.1	68.3	69.4	−0.15**
Fat	g	114.3	111.0	103.9	−0.06	85.5	82.6	93.0	−0.01
Carbohydrate	g	290.7	325.0	312.0	0.16	233.9	240.2	233.3	0.03
Calcium	mg	1138.8	1062.2	1008.2	−0.05	1085.2	883.9	962.1	−0.19**
Retinol equivalent	µg	2839.2	2318.7	2252.1	−0.17	1386.5	1097.5	1483.6	−0.01
Thiamin	mg	1.4	1.4	1.4	0.002	1.3	1.2	1.2	−0.06
Riboflavin	mg	2.0	1.9	1.8	−0.07	1.9	1.8	2.0	−0.05
Ascorbic acid	mg	115.4	86.9	92.9	−0.25**	97.3	84.1	64.0	−0.06
Nicotinic acid	mg	11.7	12.0	11.9	0.05	17.0	17.0	17.1	−0.01
Variety score		29.9	24.7	21.8	−0.43****	53.3	48.8	44.0	0.01
% Energy:									
Protein		12.6	12.6	12.6		15.3	14.4	14.3	
Fat		39.9	38.6	37.8		38.6	37.7	41.2	
CHO		45.3	48.9	49.1		45.4	47.3	44.4	

**p ≤ 0.05   ‡ Husband's occupation considered as a dichotomous variable divided between non-manual/
****p ≤ 0.001   manual occupations correlated with daily nutrient intake and variety score

Protein and fat intake contributed a similar proportion of energy in all husbands' and wives' occupational groups, while women who were in professional and clerical occupations or were the wives of non-manual workers tended to eat less carbohydrate than the rest. Correlation coefficients of energy, protein, fat and carbohydrate were not sufficiently high to be significant, which suggests that the relationship with occupations was weak.

In the 1985 survey, the women in professional and technical occupations ate most in energy, protein and fat and those in semi-skilled and unskilled occupations ate least. Using the husband's occupations trends were less evident although wives with husbands in non-manual occupations ate most protein and wives of semi-skilled and unskilled manual workers ate more fat. Correlation coefficients only reached statistical significance in respect of protein irrespective of the occupational classification used (Tables 11.8 and 11.9).

It should be stressed that in both surveys there was great variability amongst individual women in all social classes and the overlap between the occupational groups was considerable.

It may be noted that the variety score varied directly with either the woman's own or her husband's occupation in both surveys—women in professional and clerical occupations or who were the wives of non-manual workers taking a more varied diet. The differences were highly significant in 1951, but only in respect of the woman's own occupation in 1985, indicating that the wife's occupation had become more discriminating. This finding is also reinforced if minerals and vitamins are considered.

Table 11.10 shows that in the 1951 survey, the few significant associations with the wife's occupation decreased once variation in height was excluded and remained significant only for ascorbic acid. In the recent survey, the wife's occupation was independent of maternal height with significant associations remaining once the effects of height had been accounted for.

Two women in each survey produced twins and have been excluded in considering gestation and birthweight. Gestation (completed weeks) at delivery was not affected by daily dietary intake in either survey. Birthweight (Table 11.11), however, was significantly positively correlated with the main dietary items considered except for calcium, retinol equivalent and ascorbic acid in the 1951 survey, but for only fat intake in 1985. Variety of diet was not associated with birthweight in either survey. Thus, while in 1951, in general, women who ate more tended to have larger babies, in 1985 this applied only to women with a higher intake of fat. However, it is known that birthweight is positively correlated with maternal height and the existence of an association between dietary intake and the woman's height has already been described. Thus, the association noted between dietary intake and birthweight might be caused by the effect of maternal height acting jointly on dietary intake and birthweight to produce these associations. Indeed, as Table 11.12 shows, when partial correlations of dietary intake and birthweight are compared, controlling for maternal height, all coefficients are reduced and fail to be statistically significant. In comparison when

TABLE 11.10

PARTIAL CORRELATION COEFFICIENTS OF DIETARY INTAKE WITH WIFE'S OCCUPATION CONTROLLING FOR HEIGHT

	1951	1985	
	Partial correlation Height A	Partial correlation Height A	Partial correlation Height B
Energy	-0.05	-0.12	-0.03
Protein	-0.08	-0.25****	-0.14**
Fat	-0.08	-0.10	0.01
Carbohydrate	0.03	-0.04	0.004
Calcium	-0.16	-0.23***	-0.22***
Retinol equivalent	-0.17	-0.09	-0.19**
Thiamin	0.07	-0.21***	-0.03
Riboflavin	-0.12	-0.24***	-0.24***
Ascorbic acid	-0.19**	-0.22****	-0.20****
Nicotinic acid	-0.02	-0.22***	-0.19**

Dichotomous division of occupation: A Professional, technical and clerical/other
B Professional and technical/other

**p ⩽ 0.05
***p ⩽ 0.01
****p ⩽ 0.001

TABLE 11.11

MEAN DAILY NUTRIENT INTAKE, ENERGY COMPOSITION AND VARIETY SCORE BY BIRTHWEIGHT (twins excluded)

(Number)		1951				1985			
		≤2999 (25)	3000-3499 (47)	3500+ (24)	r‡	≤2999 (38)	3000-3499 (71)	3500+ (31)	r‡
Energy	MJ	10.2	10.4	11.2	0.21**	8.0	8.1	8.3	0.12
Protein	g	73.8	77.4	80.7	0.20**	69.4	69.5	73.0	0.13
Fat	g	105.5	110.0	114.2	0.18**	83.2	84.2	87.9	0.14**
Carbohydrate	g	314.9	300.6	348.6	0.20**	233.9	235.2	238.6	0.07
Calcium	mg	1061.7	1054.9	1069.6	0.09	908.9	1015.3	989.7	0.07
Retinol equivalent	µg	2303.3	2459.9	2369.9	0.08	1086.7	1347.0	1279.0	0.01
Thiamin	mg	1.3	1.4	1.6	0.21**	1.2	1.3	1.3	0.10
Riboflavin	mg	1.8	1.9	2.0	0.19**	1.8	1.9	2.0	0.07
Ascorbic acid	mg	82.3	99.2	97.1	0.16	83.5	93.2	76.1	−0.05
Nicotinic acid	mg	11.0	12.0	13.1	0.22**	17.5	16.6	18.0	−0.01
Variety score		24.9	24.9	24.9	0.03	49.3	50.3	49.6	−0.02
% energy:									
Protein		12.4	12.8	12.4		14.8	14.7	15.0	
Fat		38.2	39.2	38.0		38.2	38.4	39.0	
CHO		49.5	46.9	49.7		46.7	46.1	45.5	

‡ Correlation coefficient of nutrient intake and birthweight

**p ≤ 0.05

TABLE 11.12

PARTIAL CORRELATION COEFFICIENT OF DIETARY INTAKE WITH BIRTHWEIGHT (SINGLETONS ONLY) CONTROLLING FOR HEIGHT AND OCCUPATION

| | 1951 Partial Correlation | | | 1985 Partial Correlation | | | |
	Height	Husband's occupation‡	Wife's occupation A	Height	Husband's occupation‡	Wife's occupation A	Wife's occupation B
Energy	0.16	0.21**	0.22**	0.08	0.13	0.13	0.13
Protein	0.15	0.20**	0.21**	0.08	0.14**	0.13	0.15**
Fat	0.13	0.17	0.19**	0.10	0.14**	0.14**	0.15**
Carbohydrate	0.17	0.22**	0.21**	0.03	0.07	0.07	0.07
Calcium	0.07	0.08	0.09	-0.03	0.08	0.07	0.09
Retinol equivalent	0.08	0.07	0.08	-0.01	0.01	0.03	0.04
Thiamin	0.17	0.21**	0.23**	0.07	0.10	0.10	0.10
Riboflavin	0.17	0.18**	0.19**	0.04	0.07	0.09	0.10
Ascorbic acid	0.08	0.14	0.16	-0.05	-0.04	-0.05	-0.04
Nicotinic acid	0.16	0.22**	0.23**	-0.02	-0.01	0.01	0.02

dichotomous division of occupations: ‡ Non-manual/manual
A Professional, technical and clerical/other
B Professional and technical/other

**p ≤ 0.05

TABLE 11.13

MEAN DAILY INTAKE OF NUTRIENTS, ENERGY COMPOSITION AND VARIETY SCORE BY SMOKING

(Number)		1951			1985		
		Smoker (21)	Non-smoker (73)	r‡	Smoker (31)	Non-smoker (111)	r‡
Energy	MJ	10.7	10.5	0.05	8.3	8.1	0.04
Protein	g	79.8	76.6	0.08	69.4	70.5	-0.03
Fat	g	119.0	107.7	0.16	87.0	84.2	0.06
Carbohydrate	g	293.0	322.6	-0.16	235.8	235.6	0.001
Calcium	mg	1052.0	1073.0	-0.02	957.2	986.5	-0.02
Retinol equivalent	μg	2401.2	2326.2	-0.05	1169.7	1183.4	-0.05
Thiamin	mg	1.4	1.4	0.05	1.12	1.3	-0.13
Riboflavin	mg	1.9	1.9	-0.0005	1.7	1.9	-0.14
Ascorbic acid	mg	80.5	98.5	-0.20**	57.6	94.2	-0.21***
Nicotinic acid	mg	11.6	12.0	-0.06	15.1	17.7	-0.19**
Variety score		26.3	24.7	0.12	46.4	50.9	-0.17**
% energy:							
Protein		12.7	12.6		14.5	14.9	
Fat		40.4	38.1		39.1	38.3	
CHO		45.0	49.2		45.6	46.3	

‡ Correlation of nutrient intake and variety score with smoking
**p ⩽ 0.5
***p ⩽ 0.01

controlled for the effects of variations by occupation of the husband or wife, little change is evident in the strength of the association between dietary components and birthweight; the only difference being that protein intake in 1985 reached marginal significance for two of the three occupational classifications. Thomson (1959b) after discussing these factors and maternal weight concluded that 'the influence of diet on birthweight was small, indeed, negligible'.

About one-fifth of women in both surveys were smokers and, as a group, their diets were similar to those of non-smokers except for their lower intake of ascorbic acid (Table 11.13). In the recent study, smokers appeared to have had a less varied diet, and their intake of nicotinic acid was also lower than that of non-smokers. The small numbers and the range in the number of cigarettes smoked per day (from 1 to 40) does not permit analysis by subgroups.

MINERALS AND VITAMINS

As already noted, vitamin supplements were available free or at a nominal charge to pregnant women in the early 1950s, and in the week of their weighed survey 92 of the 94 primigravidae recorded taking these. Without supplements the mean intake fell from 1068.3 to 1019.6mg for calcium, from 1.44 to 1.40µg for thiamin, from 90.5 to 80.7mg for ascorbic acid and from 2404.5 to 2088.8µg for retinol equivalents. In marked contrast only 5 of the 142 primigravidae in the 1985 survey reported taking any such supplementation, giving a minimal overall effect. The upper limit of 644mg in the range of ascorbic acid in the recent survey (Table 11.4) is due to supplementation by one woman.

IRON AND DIETARY FIBRE

Data on intake of iron and dietary fibre was only available for the 1985 sample. The range for both was great. The present recommended daily intake of iron for pregnant women is 13mg (DHSS, 1979), whilst the primigravidae in the present study took on average 14.70mg ranging from 4 to 99mg, indicating the need for the proper diagnosis of anaemia before supplementation. The upper limit in the range is due to four women taking iron supplements.

Again, the range of dietary fibre intake varied from 3.0 to 45.4g per day, with a mean of 17.2g. This is considerably lower than the target of 25g currently recommended by the National Advisory Committee on Nutrition Education (NACNE, 1983) and only about half the longer term objective of 30g a standard met by only eight of the women.

CHAPTER 12

Summary and Comments

The 1985 study aimed at establishing whether social, dietary and obstetric factors and the associations between them had persisted or changed in 34 years. The special features of the recent study were that it was carried out by a member of the 1950s research team, in the same city which had retained a centralised maternity service covering the total population of a geographical area. The two studies, however, were carried out in very different circumstances. The first was carried out in the postwar period when families were affected by men being conscripted for National Service, and some food rationing was still in force. The recent study was conducted when the oil industry was booming, before the fall in oil prices in 1986 led to a recession in the local economy. In the intervening years the maternity services had become more centered on AMH with the decline in domiciliary service and the provision of clinics at the hospital. The general practitioner had become more involved in antenatal care, especially since the rationalisation of the antenatal services (Hall *et al.*, 1985) and in postnatal care.

The research was carried out on samples of married women whose first pregnancy ended in a birth and who resided in clearly defined local authority geographical areas (Aberdeen City in 1951, Aberdeen City District in 1985). The recent study was a very limited and streamlined version of that carried out in the early 1950s as this extended over many years and included a wealth of descriptive material. From this early experience a precoded proforma was prepared and used in 1985 to record mainly facts as reported by the women and data from the medical notes. An intensive and descriptive study of the expectations and experiences of married primigravidae in Aberdeen in the late 1970s had already been reported by Macintyre (1981).

On account of changes in social and marital behaviour indicated by unmarried motherhood and by terminations of first pregnancies under the Abortion Act 1967, the married women studied in 1985 represented a much smaller proportion of primigravidae, 60% compared with 85% in 1951. Similar changes had been taking place in other Scottish cities, in Scotland as a whole and in England and Wales. Published data show that in the intervening years Aberdeen and the Grampian Region have experienced the same trends in birth rate, stillbirths, neonatal mortality, illegitimacy and abortions under the 1967 Abortion Act as those elsewhere.

The samples can be taken as representative of the married primigravidae from whom they came. The main differences between them, thirty-four years apart, are illustrated in Figures 12.1*a*, *b* and *c*.

SOCIAL BACKGROUND

Compared with the postwar sample, the recent sample showed certain features characteristic of changes manifest throughout Britain in the intervening years as indicated by Census Reports and numerous Government publications, for example, CSO (1985). The couples were more mobile, fewer women and/or their husbands being of local origin. In-migrants were no longer so homogeneous as in the 1950s. The current sample came from smaller families, and overall more wives and husbands had been brought up by both parents. Fewer homes had been disrupted by death of a parent because of increased life expectancy and peacetime conditions, but on the other hand more parents had been separated and divorced. More couples in 1985 had fathers who were non-manual workers, reflecting changes in the industrial and occupational structure. More of the 1985 women and their husbands had stayed on at school, even though the minimum school-leaving age had been raised between the studies, and more had gone on to higher education.

Maximum height potential is genetically determined, but the association of socio-economic status and actual adult height is well known (see Knight 1984). An overall increase of about 3 cm in the mean height of women reflects the upbringing of the 1985 primigravidae in the improved postwar social environment with full employment, better working and general living conditions and the NHS.

OCCUPATIONS

The different circumstances in which the two studies were carried out had a marked effect on occupations and opportunities for employment. World War II and its aftermath had affected the working lives of nearly all the husbands and some of the wives in the 1951 sample; most of the men had been in the Armed Forces and some were still doing National Service. The recent study was carried out when the oil industry was booming. Aberdeen, from being a regional centre with declining industries such as granite, shipbuilding and fishing, had become a centre of world oil production in the 1970s. In that decade it had the highest increase in employment of any labour market in Britain and had become an importer of workers. These changes were reflected in the differences between the samples; there were more in-migrants in 1985 than in 1951 and 34% of the husbands were employed, directly or indirectly, in the oil industry. The repercussions on female employment were marked with high rates of both full-time and particularly part-time employment. The 1981 census showed that the Aberdeen North Parliamentary constituency had the highest level of part-time female employment of all constituencies in UK and the level of full-time employment was about three times higher than the national figure (Bonney, 1986).

The occupations and work histories of both the husbands and wives in the two samples reflect overall changes in education and training provision in the UK coupled with the increase in non-manual occupations and greater opportunities for employment and advancement. New industries and new technology had not only created new jobs, but revolutionised many old ones so that jobs with the same title may have been transformed. Changes in training, skill, prestige and payment may also have upset the comparative relationship of occupations at different points in time. Some of the problems of assessing socio-demographic changes by cross-sectional comparisons are discussed in the OPCS Occasional Paper 34 (1985). In the Aberdeen studies, admittedly small although representative, the problems of occupational classifications are particularly acute because of the importance in 1985 of the oil industry affecting the employment of men and because of the preponderance of wives in professional, technical and clerical occupations (73% compared with 30% in 1951) which led to re-analysis separating out the clerical workers. In general, by 1985, the wife's occupation had become more discriminating in contrast to 1951 when the husband's occupation, indicating her achieved status by marriage, was all important (Illsley, 1956a). The increased significance of the women's own occupation is also discussed by Macfarlane and Mugford (1984). This change, no doubt at least partly, reflects the opportunities now available and advancements attained by women from which so many were previously barred because of their limited education and training as well as by discrimination against women—in particular married women *per se*. The women in the recent survey were in a better position to exploit their interests and abilities. Legal protection against sex discrimination and provision of maternity leave had given the 1985 woman more choice and most (four times as many as in 1951) continued in employment not only after marriage, but during pregnancy. Although some were entitled to have their full-time job kept open for them and were advised to leave their options open, it is perhaps surprising that nearly half of eligible women in the sample said that they had not done so. Although this aspect was not studied in detail, there was some evidence that many women did not get a great deal of satisfaction or pleasure from their employment other than the social contacts and had decided to take an extended break. Baby minding did not seem to be a particular problem. Ultimately the women expected to go out to work again.

MARRIAGE AND STARTING A FAMILY

Housing developments had redistributed the population away from the congested inner-city tenement areas to outlying new housing estates. The impact of these changes was noted even in the way in which the couples in the two samples had met. In the 1980s they were more likely to have met casually 'at the disco' rather than to have known each other as neighbours in childhood.

The acute postwar housing shortage meant that most couples started their married life sharing a house, mainly with the wife's mother and particularly when pregnancy precipitated marriage there was virtually no alternative;

some engaged couples waited several years and only married when they obtained a house. Only a minority of the 1951 sample had a home of their own, which (except in the case of a few affluent couples) was usually rented in privately owned sub-standard property; even so, getting such accommodation usually depended on there being family links with a private landlord or housing factor. Most couples registered for a Council house, which they saw as their only hope of getting a home of their own, particularly one with modern conveniences. This involved waiting until they had accumulated sufficient points which were allocated for each child, overcrowding, poor facilities and medical conditions. Housing was such an overwhelming problem in the early 1950s that it was exceptional for a couple with one child to qualify for a Council house (Thompson, 1954).

The situation was totally transformed for the 1985 sample. The oil boom coupled with private house building in Aberdeen in the 1970s and early 1980s and the availability of mortgages to young men and women meant that owner-occupancy of modern houses was the norm. The changed situation is further reflected in the way in which some of the men and women had lived independently and over one-fifth had cohabited before marriage. Couples now had choice as regards location, size and type of property and also having been more geographically mobile, more had moved house.

It should not be assumed that there was no housing problem in Aberdeen in the early 1980s. Towards the end of 1985 the local papers, e.g. *Press and Journal,* 7 October 1985, highlighted concern about the increase in the waiting list for Council houses and the plight of some young newly married couples. Most couples in the 1985 sample had married before they started their planned family, they had been two income families usually until the third trimester and for some this would continue. At the time of the study they were relatively affluent, but it is likely that some of the families may later have suffered hardship following the recession in the oil industry.

Oral contraception, introduced in 1964, which has so transformed the experiences and expectations of couples, could not have been anticipated. In the earlier study most women had been fatalistic about when they started a family; overall only one in six said that they had deliberately planned their first pregnancy, and about one-quarter had conceived prenuptially. Non-use or inefficient use of contraception, mainly male methods, increased with declining occupational status. In contrast the use of contraception was almost universal in the 1985 survey and three out of four first babies were said to have been deliberately planned. Conception before marriage was exceptional, and few wives were teenagers. These women expected to control their fertility, and it may be noted that two-thirds of them were back on the pill within three months of the birth of their first child. They intended to become pregnant if and when they wished, and some couples had already decided on which partner would be sterilised in due course. Changes in contraceptive practice in Aberdeen have been part of the revolution which has occurred thorughout Britain and is well reported (e.g. Cartwright, 1978: Bone, 1980).

Asked antenatally about their family preferences the 1951 wives reported that their husbands had a marked preference for a boy; they themselves were equally divided between wanting a boy, a girl, or 'not minding'. In 1985 the emphasis for both was on having a normal, healthy child; a minority of husbands had a preference which was more likely to be for a boy. It has been suggested elsewhere (e.g., Oakley, 1980; Jackson, 1984) that it is difficult to know from responses, even of men themselves, the extent to which they really would prefer to have a son. The 1985 wives wanted fewer children and to have them closer together than their 1951 counterparts. However, in both studies two children was the most preferred family size.

THE WOMEN'S ACTIVITIES

Many primigravidae in 1951 lived with relatives or close by so that social contracts could easily be maintained. In contrast, the 1985 sample had homes of their own, often in outlying and developing suburbs at some distance from relatives. Studies from elsewhere in the early 1950s (e.g. from London, Young and Willmot, 1957) raised concern about the break up of kinship networks and the isolation of young couples in homes of their own which invariably meant at some distance from relatives. Firth and Djamour (1956), however, reported that frequency of contact and intensity in social relations were not necessarily a function of geographical proximity. In Aberdeen, contact with mothers, although less in 1985 than in 1951 when many lived in the parental home and more had mothers living locally, were still strong and maintained postnatally as also described by Macintyre (1981). About half the 1985 sample saw their mothers daily or several times a week and one quarter saw their mothers-in-law as frequently. McIntosh (1985) also reports the maintenance of close ties with relatives in similar circumstances in Glasgow. The increase in private motoring has undoubtedly been a factor in facilitating visiting. The telephone was also an important means whereby the 1985 sample kept in touch with relatives and friends as the interviewers became well aware.

The couples in 1985 had a more varied social life outside the home and the diet surveys show that they ate more snacks and meals out. More of the primigravidae took part in a wider variety of sports which were more likely to be continued into early pregnancy, especially swimming which was the most popular sport in both samples. Going to the cinema had been replaced by watching television and videos.

The 1985 primigravidae had modern well equipped homes and usually shopped infrequently at supermarkets, whereas their 1951 counterpart had either limited domestic responsibility or coped in poor conditions and shopped almost daily on foot or using public transport. Most of the 1985 sample (70%), three-and-a-half times as many as in 1951, worked for at least twenty-six weeks of pregnancy, although most were in sedentary type jobs. Whether overall the 1985 primigravidae were physically more active than those in 1951 is debatable.

DIET

The weighed diet surveys were carried out during one week, at about thirty weeks gestation, under the direction and supervision of qualified dietitians. Unfortunately, the original 1951 menus and weights recorded by the women had been destroyed and the daily intake of nutrients could not be recalculated using the same method as that for 1985. Evidence, however, indicates that doing this would probably have given very similar figures to those available.

The circumstances in 1951 were very different from those at the time of the 1985 study. Food rationing was still in force in the early 1950s, but pregnant women were allowed some extra rations, milk and vitamin supplements. Whereas 98% of the 1951 sample took vitamin supplements in the week they co-operated in the diet survey this applied to only 3.5% in 1985. Notwithstanding the activities of the Ministry of Food set up during the war and a national focus on nutrition, the dietitians found that the 1951 primigravidae had little interest in food or cooking and were very conservative in what they ate. In marked contrast, the 1985 primigravidae were very interested and often knowledgable about nutrition and were concerned about taking a 'good diet' and the implications for their baby and their own longterm health. More of them provided a complete and reliable record of their diet, 92% compared with 80% in 1951 when it must be remembered that some women had found it difficult to co-operate when they were boarding or sharing facilities in sublet accommodation.

The indications overall are that the 1985 primigravidae may have eaten less in energy than those in 1951, but they had a more varied diet. They derived a significantly higher proportion of energy from protein and less from carbohydrates than their 1951 counterparts; the proportion derived from fats was similar in the two samples.

The recent study confirmed some associations with daily nutrient intake found in the 1951 diet surveys.

1 Overall, diets high in one nutrient were likely to be high in others.
2 Maternal height: shorter women ate less than taller women which could not be accounted for by occupational status. The proportion of energy derived from protein, fat and carbohydrate did not vary with height groups.
3 Smoking: one-fifth of primigravidae in each sample smoked. Smokers had a similar diet to non-smokers except for a significant reduction in ascorbic acid.
4 Birthweight: although in 1951 women who ate more in energy tended to have heavier babies, this tendency disappeared when controlled for height and was little affected by occupational status. It was concluded that dietary intake, as measured, had little or no influence on birthweight. This was confirmed by the 1985 study. There was also no association between birthweight and variety score in either study.
5 Variety score: in both studies women who were professional, technical or

clerical workers had a significantly more varied diet than women in other occupational groups. This also applied to wives of non-manual workers in 1951, but not in 1985, indicating that by then the woman's own occupation had become more discriminating.

The relationship between the components of energy and occupational groups was weak in 1951 although wives of semi-skilled and unskilled manual workers or women who were in similar low status occupations themselves tended to eat the most carbohydrate. These male and female occupational groups in 1985 showed a significantly lower intake of energy from protein compared with other occupational groups, but the wife's occupation was more discriminating. In both samples there was great variability in diets and a considerable overlap between diets in the different occupational groups.

The contribution of vitamins and other items to the diets analysed was variable and is considered in Chapter 9.

DELIVERY AND OUTCOME

The increasing medicalisation of and obstetric intervention in childbirth has been well publicised. Not unexpectedly, therefore, these developments were evident when the experiences of the 1951 and 1985 samples were compared.

The 1985 deliveries were more concentrated around term and two-and-a-half times as many of the women had labour induced. The proportion of spontaneous deliveries had fallen from three-quarters in 1951 to one-half in 1985—both caesarean section and forceps deliveries had markedly increased and this also applied to episiotomies.

More women were recorded as having all types of pre-eclampsia in 1985 and although the same definition was applied as in 1951 (Nelson, 1955) there may have been more regular monitoring of blood pressure especially during labour. It was later in the 1950s that significant findings on the behaviour of blood pressure during labour were being reported. More women in the 1985 sample were also affected by antepartum haemorrhage, a condition the causes of which remain obscure, whereas fewer suffered from postpartum haemorrhage which may be averted by medication. Prediction of complications and abnormalities although improved in certain areas, e.g. screening for certain genetic conditions, has largely continued to be baffling and clinical practice is largely empirical. Also the scientific understanding of the fundamental biological and physiological processes of pregnancy and birth remains fairly primitive, e.g. what triggers off labour.

A spectacular rise in fetal distress recorded in the obstetric records, 83% compared with 18% in 1951, undoubtedly exaggerates the situation and implicates the new technology of continuous fetal monitoring and the varied criteria for ascertainment. The diagnosis was seldom a matter of real concern and it was reported to few women as a cause for action.

Nearly all the 1985 women had some medication to alleviate the pain of childbirth compared with less than two-thirds in 1951. Also nearly half the 1985 sample, over twice as many as in 1951, had an epidural performed, although fewer had a general anaesthetic.

The outcome presents a paradox as perinatal mortality and birthweight (distribution and mean) were similar in the two samples. To avoid possible confounding physiological factors both studies had been restricted to first pregnancies. Some improvements in outcome might have been expected because the 1985 women were taller and fewer were teenagers, nearly all the babies had been planned and there had been revolutionary improvements in socio-economic conditions. Smoking is known to be a hazard, but a similar proportion of women in each sample were smokers and pregnancy did not influence the habit.

The marked overall fall in perinatal mortality over the years is described in Chapter 2, but is not reflected in these relatively small samples. Fraser (1983) in a literature review of the scientific basis for use and psychosocial effects of certain perinatal procedures has questioned the use of mortality as a gauge of successful intervention and stressed the need for randomised controlled trials to clarify the benefits and hazards of certain obstetric practices. She also noted the chain reaction in the chance of procedures being applied and the neglect of long-term follow-up to assess the implications of obstetric interventions. She concluded that the obstetric procedures considered were not pleasant to the majority of women but were tolerated if believed to be necessary. The failure of birthweight to rise has become a matter of national concern as low birthweight is a powerful predictor of infant death (OPCS, 1986) and has important implications for physical and intellectual development (Fraser, 1984). Although some associations have been well established, e.g. with smoking, social disadvantage and problems, the aetiology of birthweight remains elusive. An interesting finding in Aberdeen is that in the case of twins, whereas the birthweight of twins I over the years has behaved like that of singletons, that of twin II has increased significantly so that overall twins born in the 1980s are of fairly similar weight, the previous birthweight disadvantage of twin II having disappeared (Campbell and Samphier, 1988).

Various explanations have been suggested to explain the failure of birthweight to rise.

A genetic contribution to reproduction efficiency cannot be discounted as genetic inheritance sets certain limits, e.g. potential adult height. Carr-Hill et al., (1987) in a three generational family study using Aberdeen data compared the birthweights of the first born to grandmothers and to their daughters: the correlation coefficients were somewhat less than those reported for cousins (Robson, 1955) and they concluded that genetics made only a small contribution to birthweight. Billewicz (1972), however, considered that a first birth was not necessarily typical of a woman's reproduction because of the special risks involved, e.g. pre-eclampsia, and discounted primiparae in an analysis of the birthweights of full siblings. He showed the importance of different philosophical approaches in the method of standardisation used in the analysis. A good prediction of a woman having a low birthweight baby is her previous history of producing such lightweight babies (Carr-Hill *et al.*, 1987) which is irrelevant for primiparae. Ounsted *et al.*, (1988) found that the percentage of low birthweight babies more than doubled if the mothers themselves reported that they had been of low birthweight. In considering any genetic contribution the father cannot be ignored. For example, Sutherland (1980) suggested that gestation length was under parental control. Also it has been shown that previous preterm delivery is the best predictor of a preterm birth (Illsley and Thompson, 1976) and there was a familial pattern in pre-eclampsia (Adams and Finlayson, 1961). It is of interest that Blaxter (1982) in her study of family health noted that mothers gave hereditary factors more importance than is usually acknowledged by professionals.

Whereas genetics 'may set limitations' the end result will depend on the pervasive social and environmental factors mediated through the woman's physiological efficiency in adapting to pregnancy. In considering the relative stability of birthweight over time a neglected area of research is the importance of the woman's level of activity and how this affects her health and physiology. Lifestyles have changed markedly, but the changes in physical activity are uncertain. Some attention has focused on employment during pregnancy (e.g. Chamberlain, 1984). However, records in Aberdeen in the 1950s indicated that the paid work undertaken by a minority of women during pregnancy was not detrimental (Illsley, *et al.*, 1954). As already reported in the 1980s most women worked into the third trimester, but the actual work they did and the environmental conditions had changed.

Certainly strenuous physical activity may have a deleterious effect on the fetus because of impaired blood flow to the uterus (Hytten, 1984) and should be avoided. Some French studies (Mammele and Laumon, 1984) have suggested that fatigue as measured by factors such as posture, machine work, repetitive gestures, etc., may lead to preterm delivery. Before World War II it was reported that the birthweight of babies born to textile workers was depressed when the women stood rather than sat at work (Balfour, 1938). The questions that have to be answered are first, whether doing paid work during pregnancy carries greater risk to pregnancy outcome than staying at home and secondly, what should be the limitations on activity: If causative factors are to be identified then in-depth studies of physical, chemical, biological and psycho-social factors will be necessary and the different stresses balanced against each other, e.g. the loss of income and what that entails against change in physical activity. Factors to be considered would include pollution in relation to toxicity and radiation in the environment whether at home or work which might affect the fetus, subliminal noises and maternal activity. The possible relevance of the husband's working environment might also be considered. Although the Aberdeen diet survey shows that birthweight is not dependent upon diet as measured this does not preclude the possibility of some aspect of diet being important, such as particular items or the balance between them, but current evidence tends to discount this. We need to know the scientific facts and until causative factors rather than associations can be identified little progress will be made and it will be difficult to advise individual women. Also, a study of low birthweight (Illsley and Mitchell, 1984) concluded that research was needed to define normality by establishing precisely what is meant by a baby being born at appropriate size for a given maternal conformation and progress during pregnancy. This same study showed that certain perinatal disadvantages could be overcome if the child was brought up in a good environment. It should also be noted that Carr-Hill and Pritchard (1988) argue that birthweight standards for clinical use must be derived from local populations.

POSTNATAL EXPERIENCES

Differences between the samples in problems in the puerperium and later reflect changes in hospital policy on breast feeding and increased medical and obstetric intervention.

One-fifth of each sample had problems in the puerperium according to the medical records, but these did not include some conditions which were distressing and painful to the women and for which treatment may have been given. Improvements in general health and medical advances were demonstrated in 1985 by the absence of active tuberculosis and the need for transfer for various conditions to the infectious diseases hospital. In both studies, infection of the urinary tract was the commonest problem in the puerperium, although less frequent in 1985. The women had a significantly shorter stay in hospital in 1985—mean 6.3 days compared with 8.8 days in 1951.

More primiparae in 1985 reported health problems arising at home in the 13 weeks following delivery—half compared with one-third in 1951. To some extent this difference may reflect the greater readiness of the better educated, more articulate and independent women in the mid 1980s, who had always known the NHS, to seek advice more readily, particularly about gynaecological problems. There were major differences, however, in the problems reported.

In 1951 when breast feeding in AMH was mandatory, problems with breasts and in suppressing lactation were dominant, but in 1985 when women had a choice on breast feeding, such problems were exceptional. The way in which the policy of a maternity hospital went against the wishes and inclinations of a significant number of women had consequences for the general hospital as well as for general practitioners is well illustrated by these two samples.

In 1985 problems reflected the greater obstetric intervention and included anaesthetic sequelae and in particular infections of abdominal and perineal wounds and stitches.

The proportion of mothers—one in ten—who 'did not feel fully recovered' three months after the birth was similar in the two samples.

Although there have been considerable developments in antenatal care since the early 1950s, little attention has been given to the postnatal period. In the early 1970s the bonding of mother and baby became a topical subject and more recently attention has focused on the father's role. The maternity and child welfare services have always focused on the baby.

A national assessment of postnatal care is long overdue. The objectives and duration of various sections of care, e.g. hospital stay, are not defined. Account would need to be taken of women with different obstetric experiences and in different social circumstances, and what they want. Consideration of postnatal morbidity should identify iatrogenic problems and lead to recommendations for possible prevention.

The Aberdeen studies have shown how the increased involvement of general practitioners and the reorganisation of health visitors have improved the support and care within the community. However, the relevance of patterns of care as at present shared and provided to different risk groups needs to be critically assessed in the interests of the health and wellbeing of mothers and of the efficiency of the hospital and community services.

The Baby

The vast majority of the babies—eight or nine out of ten—were rated as in excellent or very good condition at birth, although by different methods of assessment. Fewer babies in 1985 were admitted to the Special Nursery and they stayed a shorter time so that more were able to go home with their mothers. Nearly half the 1985 mothers and babies were discharged together from AMH in under six days; such a short stay was exceptional in 1951. On average the neonates spent three days less in hospital in 1985 than in 1951.

The feeding experience of the babies was different in that 26% of the 1985 sample were never put to the breast compared with 2% in 1951, indicating the change in hospital policy. More women abandoned breast feeding in AMH in 1985 than in 1951. For some women breast feeding was by no means the easy and pleasant experience they had anticipated and most found that initially it produced considerable anxiety. Some mothers require a good deal of help and encouragement from nurses in order to breast feed successfully. Receiving such attention in the 1980s could present difficulties as the AMH staff were hard pressed in dealing with one and a half times as many deliveries as officially allowed for (Templeton, 1986). Many mothers in 1951 when AMH insisted on breast feeding, gave up immediately or soon after discharge incurring problems as discussed earlier. More mothers in 1985 than in 1951 blamed problems with the baby not fixing or slow feeding for stopping breast feeding. Notwithstanding the initial differences in experience by thirteen weeks, 38% of babies in each sample were being breast fed, antenatal intention and motivation being the most important factors in continuing.

The giving of solids, particularly to artificially fed babies has become widespread throughout the country and in 1985, Aberdeen was no exception. Why and how this has developed since the 1950s is uncertain. The women knew the official recommendation, but did not seem to know the reason for it and the giving of solids before 3-4 months was a bone of contention between the mothers and health visitors.

More babies in the 1985 sample were reported to have had health problems for which they attended the Children's Hospital or the general practitioner (71% compared with 58% in 1951). A similar proportion had been in hospital; two 1951 babies had been admitted with fractures following accidents in poor, overcrowded homes. Attendance at outpatient clinics in 1985 was inflated by routine follow-up for neonatal conditions noted in AMH, e.g. clicking hips. The general practitioner only had been consulted about most problems, predominantly colds and chest infections in both studies; otherwise the emphasis was somewhat different being related to breast feeding in 1951, but to colic, sticky eyes and rashes in 1985. The 1985 mothers had known the NHS throughout their lives, and living on their own and being more independent, were more likely to consult their general practitioner about fairly minor problems: the numbers might well have been greater without the Health Visitors Emergency Call Service (see below). The change in general practice from a home visiting to a surgery consultation service is clearly demonstrated.

PARTICIPATION OF HUSBANDS

There had been a cultural revolution in the involvement of husbands between the studies. In the 1950s acceptance of the separate roles of men and women was the rule. Husbands were expected to be the family wage-earners and responsible for contraception. Most primigravidae saw themselves as housewives and mothers in the foreseeable future and the idea of returning to work was hardly considered other than possibly 'in the fish' where hours were variable and family members co-operated in keeping jobs open for each other. As far as the study was concerned the husbands were shadowy figures in the background apart from a few who helped with the diet survey.

The access of husbands to AMH was strictly controlled and any suggestion that they attended the birth would have been considered indecent. Domestic help was not expected from them and the shared or cramped housing conditions did not encourage it; any help they gave was usually kept secret from relatives and friends, to avoid embarrassment or ridicule. Postnatally, most fathers did little more than occasionally nurse the baby and regular help with baby care was exceptional in the first three months. A few fathers might like to have been more involved, but were discouraged by the help given by female relatives, usually the wife's mother, with whom the couple shared a house. Husbands were never expected to take sole responsibility for the baby and would not have been competent to do so.

The situation was quite changed in the 1980s. Almost without exception the wives now took responsibility for contraception. Most continued to be wage earners during pregnancy and expected to resume employment in the future. Most couples had a home of their own, but the traditional organisation of household and domestic tasks continued with women seemingly accepting the situation without criticism (Macintyre, 1981) as also reported from elsewhere (e.g. Martin and Roberts, 1984). The husbands, however, were expected to take an active part in preparing for fatherhood. They were specifically included in antenatal and parenthood classes and their presence in the labour ward was regarded as natural and desirable. Unlike their 1951 counterparts, they were familiar with the process of childbirth and possible complications from the media, particularly from television. Most husbands volunteered enthusiastically to accompany their wives during labour and delivery. Some of the wives, however, admitted that husbands were under pressure; while they were understanding and sympathetic to husbands who might feel apprehensive or squeamish, they said that the pressures from workmates and peers made it difficult for fathers not to conform and be present in the labour ward. Most husbands were said to have found it a rewarding experience and felt 'cheated' if, for medical reasons, they were unable to witness the birth. It was commonplace for the husband to take time off work when his wife and baby were discharged from AMH, thus taking over the role which in earlier days the wife's mother had usually filled. By the time the baby was three months old, most mothers thought the fathers were competent in baby care, although many remained apprehensive about bathing the baby.

The involvement of the husbands in 1985 could not have been envisaged by those in 1951. In the second edition of his influential manual *Baby and Child Care* Spock (1958) felt it necessary to assert the possibility of being a 'warm father and real man at the same time'. In 1966 a Leader in the *Lancet* questioned the motives of husbands who wished to be present in the labour ward and stressed the complications this would make for the staff. It stated: 'For many husbands the reality of labour may be a disturbing experience and it is asking a lot of them to expect that they will bring much comfort to their wives. To be emotionally involved in the situation is also a disadvantage for this affects judgement.' It goes on to exhort that little attention should be paid 'to the vociferous minority who see nothing but good in husbands sharing the labour experience'.

Until the 1970s husbands or partners were seldom mentioned in the relevant literature as all attention focused on the mother antenatally and on the baby postnatally. Sociologists studying motherhood began increasingly to consider the father's position (e.g. Richman and Goldthorpe, 1978; Oakley, 1979, 1980; McKee, 1980) and some studies focused on fathers in their own right (e.g. Jackson, 1984). Spock in his fourth edition (1979) was advocating 'the need of the father's full participation in the care of the baby and in the housework'.

The revolutionary cultural change in the husband's participation as reported from Aberdeen is a general phenomenon occurring at different rates in different areas and sub-groups of the population throughout the country. The experience of the 1985 Aberdeen sample was very similar to that reported from Swansea (Cleary and Shepperdson, 1981*a* and *b*), another city with a large core of local families. The South Wales study, however, included couples who were unmarried and rather more who retained traditional views of the separate roles of men and women. As in Aberdeen, fathers helped postnatally notwithstanding the availability of female relatives and a close kin network. Oakley (1979) postulated, however, that the birth produces a peak of masculine domesticity and this declines as the baby grows older.

We know of no longitudinal study on the effects of the father's attendance at the birth and his early involvement with the baby. Experience of and reactions to childbirth by fathers as by mothers are very varied as indicated in Aberdeen and are often not concordant for the couple (see Appendix). Undoubtedly some husbands may participate under pressure and it may be alien for them to be involved in what they have been brought up to consider as 'strictly for women'. The shared experience according to Aberdeen mothers, was important in bonding the family together. However, the consequences for the marriage, the family and ultimately for society, of the involvement of husbands or partners in the new pattern of fatherhood needs further research.

It is unlikely that the attendance of husbands/partners in labour wards would have become so popular if the consequences to staff and labour management foreshadowed in the *Lancet* Leader (1966) had been widespread, but the costs and benefits merit investigation.

USE OF SERVICES

The antenatal, postnatal and child welfare services had been reorganised between the studies. In the 1950s antenatal care and the postnatal examination were the responsibility of the hospital although some clinics were held in local authority premises where child welfare services were provided. Obstetricians with the help of local authority medical officers, staffed the antenatal and postnatal clinics. Child welfare and the family planning clinics were the responsibility of the local authority. A private family planning clinic had recently been taken over by the local authority and established in the basement of the main antenatal clinic which was in the centre of the city and not at AMH.

By 1984 all family medical care was centred on general practices to which health visitors were now attached. Antenatal care was usually shared between the hospital where the main clinic was now situated, and general practitioners, under a new rationalised scheme (Hall et al., 1985). Unless there had been obstetric problems, general practitioners undertook most postnatal care and the child welfare services. With the introduction of the pill and IUCD general practitioners had the main responsibility for contraception, although a minority of women attended the family planning clinic, now reorganised within the NHS.

The need for a referral by a general practitioner and the introduction of an appointments system accounted for the later first attendance at the ANC of the 1985 sample, notwithstanding the decline in prenuptial conceptions, a factor associated with late attendance (Illsley, 1956b; McKinlay, 1970).

Fatalistic attitudes, common in the 1950s had virtually disappeared by 1985. Few 1951 women took advantage of the limited antenatal classes provided, preferring 'not to know' what childbirth might involve or relying on lay sources of information, especially mothers, who had often been confined at home. The 1985 sample had more knowledge of childbearing from the media, especially TV and from women's magazines and specific literature, but most attended the antenatal classes which were planned to include husbands. In both studies, women who attended particularly welcomed the classes for the opportunities they provided for fostering friendships and social support. They also 'wanted to do right' but accepted what was provided with little questioning as found by (Macintyre, 1981).

Unlike the 1985 women, many women in the 1951 study did not attend for postnatal examination. This applied especially to those in the lower occupational groups who seemed dominated by mothers who scorned 'all the fuss' being made about childbearing and did not encourage their daughters, who often lived with them, to take advantage of facilities provided. Mothers whose own experience of childbearing was prior to the NHS were not orientated towards preventive medicine. Many of the young primiparae were also deterred by extreme modesty although there was some evidence that if they had definite gynaecological problems they preferred the anonymity of the hospital to attending their GP.

In both periods the women were discharged from hospital into the care of midwives until the statutory designated 10 days postnatally had expired. After this time the health visitors kept the women and their babies under supervision by regular home visits, less frequent if the women attended the child welfare clinic. The effectiveness of the health visitors depended on the primiparae's independence and receptivity, her knowledge and experience in baby care and the rapport established. Many women in the earlier study resented the health visitors whom they looked on as 'snoopers'. The attitude to health visitors in Aberdeen in the early 1950s was very similar to that reported among working class first time mothers in Glasgow in the late 1970s (McIntosh, 1985) where surveillance and social control were thought to be their duties. Although visits might be appreciated socially and there was seldom antipathy towards an individual health visitor, nevertheless they were resented as primarily identified with child neglect and maternal incompetence.

In contrast, most women in the 1985 study welcomed the visits from the health visitor for the reassurance and opportunities for advice they gave. They were also appreciated in helping to relieve the isolation of women living alone at home at some distance from relatives. The attachment of the service to general practices in more recent years had helped understanding of the role of health visitors, who had actually been seen making a contribution to health education and conducting clinics in collaboration with GPs. However, as time went on the 1985 women sometimes found contacts with health visitors embarrassing: the widespread practice of feeding solids before 3-4 months especially to bottle fed babies was a matter of contention. The women behaved empirically and generally seemed unaware of the reasons behind the recommendation to delay giving solids. Blaxter and Paterson (1982) have reported on the difficulties encountered by Aberdeen health visitors in combating early feeding of solids, which was not a feature in 1951.

The practice and the problems it raises with health visitors is very widespread. McIntosh (1985) reported that 74% of the Glasgow primiparae he studied had given solids before their babies were twelve weeks old. A Working Party on Infant Feeding of the Committee on Medical Aspects of Food Policy (HMSO, 1979) which accepted that a flexible approach was desirable reported:

> We agree that the age at which solid foods are introduced into the diet should be individually determined from a consideration of the method of feeding practised, the developmental progress of the baby and the preference of the mother. It seems likely that the majority of infants should be offered a mixed diet not later than the age of six months and that very few will require solid foods before the age of three months.

An important innovation by the health visitors has been the introduction of a 24-hour emergency telephone advice service: a call is usually followed by a home visit. Nearly all the 1985 primiparae had a telephone and nearly half used the service, while others said that knowing that advice was so readily available had given them confidence. The women were concerned to know when it was appropriate to call the GP; in fact this was only advised to one-sixth of the mothers who used the emergency service. Most enquiries were about commonly occurring, but stressful, situations, e.g. baby sleeping fitfully or crying excessively, about which little information or advice is given in the literature or media (Graham, 1979).

All the 1985 primiparae had taken their baby to the child welfare clinic and they had gone more frequently than the 80% in the earlier sample who attended. The reorganisation of this service based on general practices, so that clinics were often in surgeries or health centres had encouraged the women who knew that if there was any problem their own GP or the on-duty practice doctor would be available immediately, whereas in the early 1950s with clinics located and run independently by the local authority a referral would have been necessary. In both periods, however, the women said that they attended primarily in order to have the baby weighed. Some women in the earlier sample preferred to have this done at a chemist's shop without undressing the baby; at that time 'a good chemist' was an important source of medical help for some lower social class families.

In 1951, the few women who used the diaphragm attended the family planning clinic and paid for the device; general practitioners were not involved. In the 1960s, the use of contraception was revolutionised by new techniques under medical control. In 1985, contraception was free within the NHS and in Aberdeen young women overwhelmingly favoured the pill. Most of the 1985 sample had obtained supplies through their general practitioner, but a minority preferred to attend the family planning clinic for reasons of convenience, greater anonymity or preference for the detailed examination routinely made there.

In general, changes in the use of services by the two samples could be accounted for by various factors including the reorganisation of services based on general practices with health visitor attachment, technological advances, changes in social behaviour and improved knowledge and independence of the women.

SOCIAL SELECTION AND OCCUPATION

In the 1950s when the late Sir Dugald Baird pioneered research in social obstetrics and gynaecology, research concentrated on married primigravidae and the association between the husbands' occupations. i.e. social class, and maternal, social and physical characteristics and obstetric outcome. At that time the immediate aim was the prevention of 'obstetric deaths' i.e. still-births and early deaths. As the research proceeded in the different areas, e.g. nutrition, physical and intellectual development, physiological adaptation to pregnancy and obstetric experience and outcome, all factors were considered in relation to social characteristics. For example, it was found that women in both upper and lower social classes had a high rate of caesarean section, but the reasons for such intervention were different—in the upper social classes the women tended to marry late and were past the best physiological age to start childbearing, whereas in the lower social classes the women although younger were of short stature and likely to have a contracted pelvis due to being brought up in conditions of poverty; the few upper social class women who were of similar short stature did not have such pelvic deformities as confirmed by a limited research project which included X-ray pelvimetries.

The sociological research also looked at the composition of the occupational groups, their characteristics and behaviour, the significance of migration as well as exclusion by definition, e.g. unmarried mothers. Studies of social mobility revealed selection factors operating which served to perpetuate and reinforce differences, e.g. the upwardly mobile women were more likely to come from smaller families, be taller, have higher intelligence test scores and lower perinatal mortality than those they left behind and the opposite applied for the downwardly mobile. The timing of marriage and of having a first baby were markedly different between the social classes or women's occupational groups: amongst married women prenuptial conception (one quarter) was associated with low social status, but the unmarried had the lowest status of all; those who married before their first pregnancy (comparable to almost the entire 1985 sample) were the most advantaged.

Many experiences in Aberdeen as revealed by the various analyses conducted in the course of the comparative study of primigravidae in 1951 and 1985, have been similar to overall national trends (CSO, 1985). These included: increase in those staying on at school; a decline in teenage marriage and prenuptial conception; about one quarter of first marriages of both partners follows a period of cohabitation; an increase in single women having abortions and also in illegitimacy; more non-manual workers and more economically active women; an increase in owner occupancy and improved housing facilities and standards; more access to private cars and the popularity of swimming; a shorter average stay in a maternity hospital.

However, the studies did not show a decrease in perinatal mortality which had occurred in the total Aberdeen population and nationally; nor had the proportion of smokers declined. Birthweight was very similar in the two samples and had been remarkably stable over time.

Two major innovations occurred between the studies, the pill introduced in 1964 and the Abortion Act 1967, of which the higher occupational groups readily availed themselves; the other groups with declining status showed a much slower acceptance of these provisions, the lowest social group lagging well behind (Thompson, 1977). These innovations affected the proportion of primigravidae available for selection to the sample in 1985. By definition the married women whose first pregnancy had ended in abortion, mostly terminations of pregnancy under the Act, were excluded. Also excluded was a much higher proportion of unmarried, first pregnancy, primigravidae than in 1951, most of whom were cohabiting with an unmarried partner; this is a general and increasing phenomenon (Brown and Kiernan, 1981) and indicates a new pattern of parenthood in view of the fact that since the introduction of the pill, fatalism about becoming a parent seems to have largely disappeared. Nevertheless, Samphier and Cunningham-Burley, (1987) in an analysis of recent Aberdeen data, have shown marked social and obstetric selection factors in six marital status groups based on legal status and cohabitation—the group from which the 1985 sample came being the most advantaged. Furthermore, they found that within each marital status category there was an independent occupational gradient from the highest, most advantaged, to the lowest, most disadvantaged, in a range of social, obstetric and perinatal factors studied.

Although the 1985 primigravidae were more homogeneous than those in 1951, similar gradients in occupational status differences persisted notwithstanding marked overall advantages such as increase in mean height, concentration of age in the 20s and planned babies. For many factors, however, the wife's own occupation had become more significant in 1985 than that of her husband, but the classification used was important, in some cases only revealing a trend when clerical workers were separated from professional and technical workers; however, this did not always apply as the clerical group had the fewest tall women. This finding on the wife's occupation is important, particularly in view of the increasing incidence of unmarried motherhood.

Most of the associations between social class and childbearing have become well established (Butler and Bonham, 1963; Macfarlane and Mugford, 1984; Health Education Council, 1987) and the Black Report (DHSS, 1980) dealt with inequalities in health in general. Social class is only a social construct and a surrogate for a variety of attributes such as education and training, cultural attitudes, material possessions and 'life style'. Constant reiteration of associations does remarkably little to advance knowledge and the severe limitations of this approach are well discussed by (Blaxter, 1980).

Illsley (1980) in a historical review of differential changes in response to premarital first pregnancy by occupational groups commented:

At the societal level, we are still unclear about the structural origins of such remarkable changes in sexual mores, courtship patterns, and reproductive behaviour in teenagers and young persons. Most major changes in social behaviour affecting large sections of society do have their origins in economic and technological developments, but they can only be traced by understanding their subjective meaning to individuals whose separate actions, when aggregated, constitute a social movement. Unfortunately sociologists were rather rare in the 1950s and 1960s and family sociology had a low status in the profession at that time so that the basic observations on which sound theory could be built were never made.

This is a legacy which presents a challenge to present day sociologists to concentrate on attempting to understand the processes by which the interaction of structural and individual social factors are translated into health, obstetric experience and outcome.

This monograph has given an account of the social, dietary and obstetric experience of a clearly defined, albeit decreasing, subgroup of married primigravidae in 1951 and 1985 in one Scottish city with a unified obstetric service. Marital and pregnancy behaviour in Aberdeen largely reflects changes which have occurred throughout Britain in the intervening years. The monograph highlights some of the neglected areas of knowledge and others where new and imaginative approaches are required.

Undoubtedly lifestyle and the environment affect development and general health, but their specific relationship to reproductive performance is largely obscure. Although much progress has been made in identifying associated factors, there has been little advance in establishing cause and effect. The married women studied were representative of the most socially advantaged primigravidae and the 1985 sample was particularly advantaged compared with the 1951 sample and significantly taller, nevertheless these advantages were not reflected in improved reproductive performance. Crudely differentiated subgroups continued to be identified by different patterns of social and obstetric experience. The problem is complex and understanding is restricted by the relative dearth of well substantiated data on the contribution of genetics and physiology. To some extent what is 'normal' has been obscured by the medicalisation of pregnancy and childbirth in Western society. Also, in order to understand some aspects, e.g. the possible influence of diet, it is necessary to go outside affluent communities e.g. Prentice and Prentice (1988). Much research is required to determine the factors fundamental to efficient childbearing. It may be that the contribution of different factors in the components of genetic, physiological, social, environmental and psychological influences are of limited importance in their own right and only become significant in their cumulative or interactive effect. Knowing the answers has important implications for targeting areas for education and the most efficient use of resources, but more importantly for giving mothers as pleasurable an experience of childbirth as possible and in giving all children the best possible start in life.

FIGURE 12.1 a SOME SIGNIFICANT PERCENTAGE DIFFERENCES BETWEEN 1951 AND 1985 SAMPLES

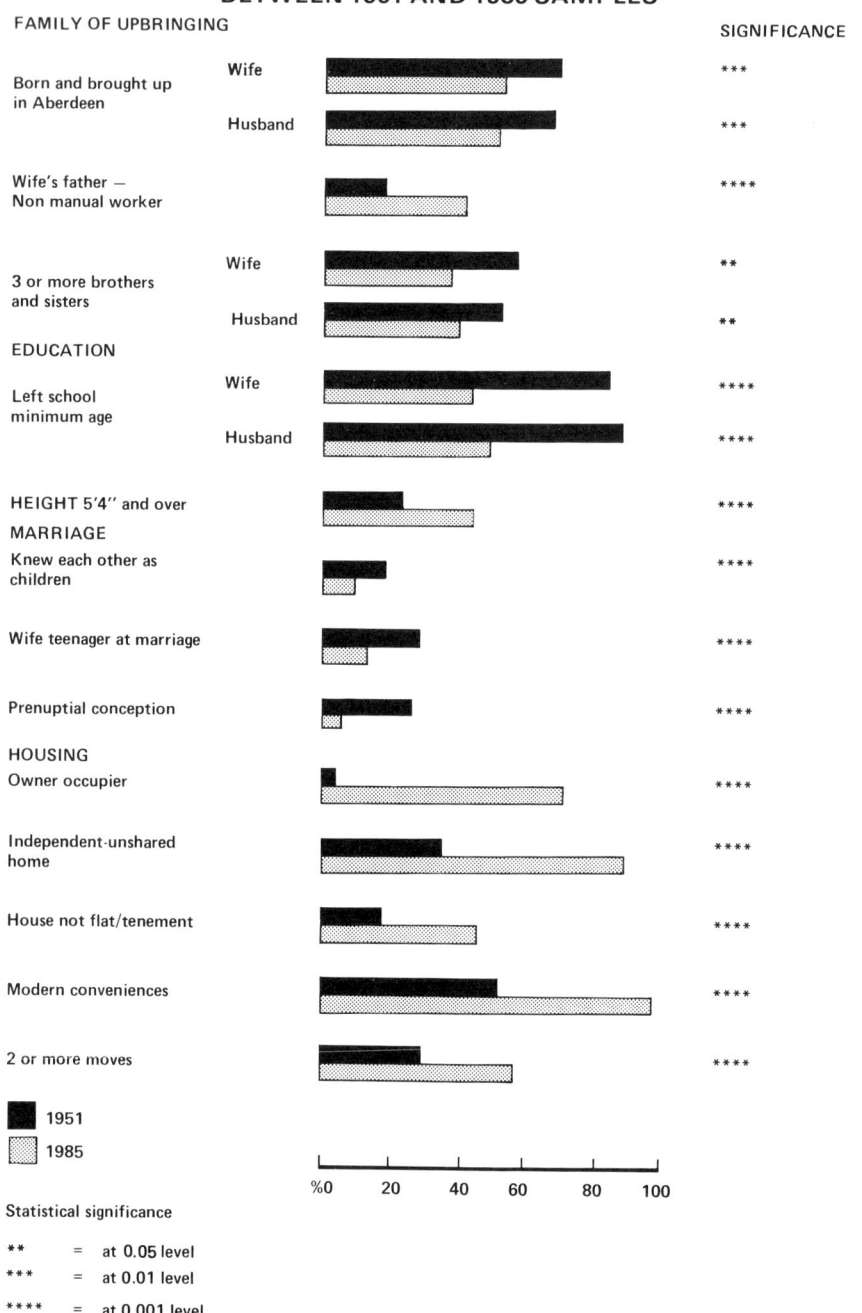

FAMILY OF UPBRINGING

SIGNIFICANCE

Born and brought up in Aberdeen — Wife — ***
Husband — ***

Wife's father — Non manual worker — ****

3 or more brothers and sisters — Wife — **
Husband — **

EDUCATION

Left school minimum age — Wife — ****
Husband — ****

HEIGHT 5'4" and over — ****

MARRIAGE

Knew each other as children — ****

Wife teenager at marriage — ****

Prenuptial conception — ****

HOUSING

Owner occupier — ****

Independent-unshared home — ****

House not flat/tenement — ****

Modern conveniences — ****

2 or more moves — ****

■ 1951

▨ 1985

%0   20   40   60   80   100

Statistical significance

**   =   at 0.05 level
***   =   at 0.01 level
**** =   at 0.001 level

FIGURE 12.1 b SOME SIGNIFICANT PERCENTAGE DIFFERENCES BETWEEN 1951 AND 1985 SAMPLES

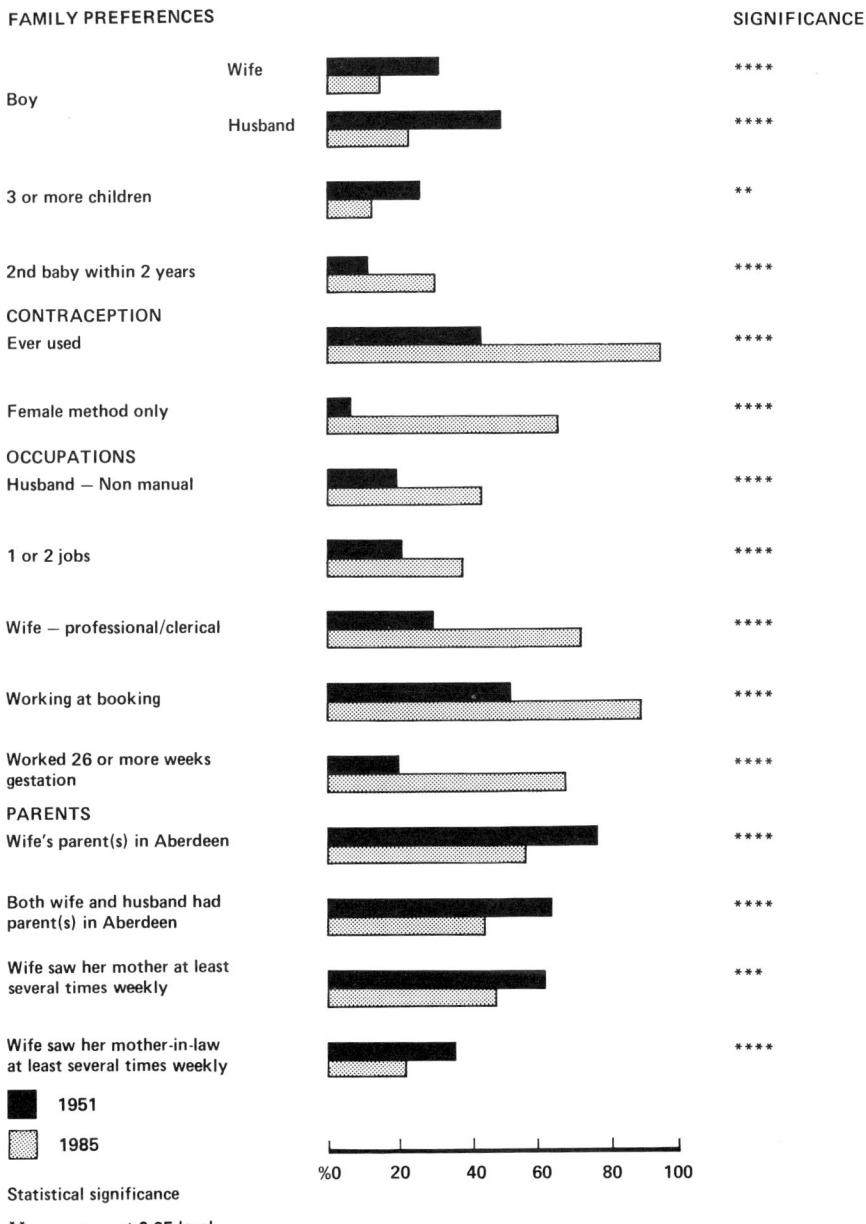

FAMILY PREFERENCES   SIGNIFICANCE

Boy — Wife ★★★★

Boy — Husband ★★★★

3 or more children ★★

2nd baby within 2 years ★★★★

CONTRACEPTION
Ever used ★★★★

Female method only ★★★★

OCCUPATIONS
Husband — Non manual ★★★★

1 or 2 jobs ★★★★

Wife — professional/clerical ★★★★

Working at booking ★★★★

Worked 26 or more weeks gestation ★★★★

PARENTS
Wife's parent(s) in Aberdeen ★★★★

Both wife and husband had parent(s) in Aberdeen ★★★★

Wife saw her mother at least several times weekly ★★★

Wife saw her mother-in-law at least several times weekly ★★★★

■ 1951

▦ 1985

%0   20   40   60   80   100

Statistical significance

★★   =   at 0.05 level

★★★   =   at 0.01 level

★★★★   =   at 0.001 level

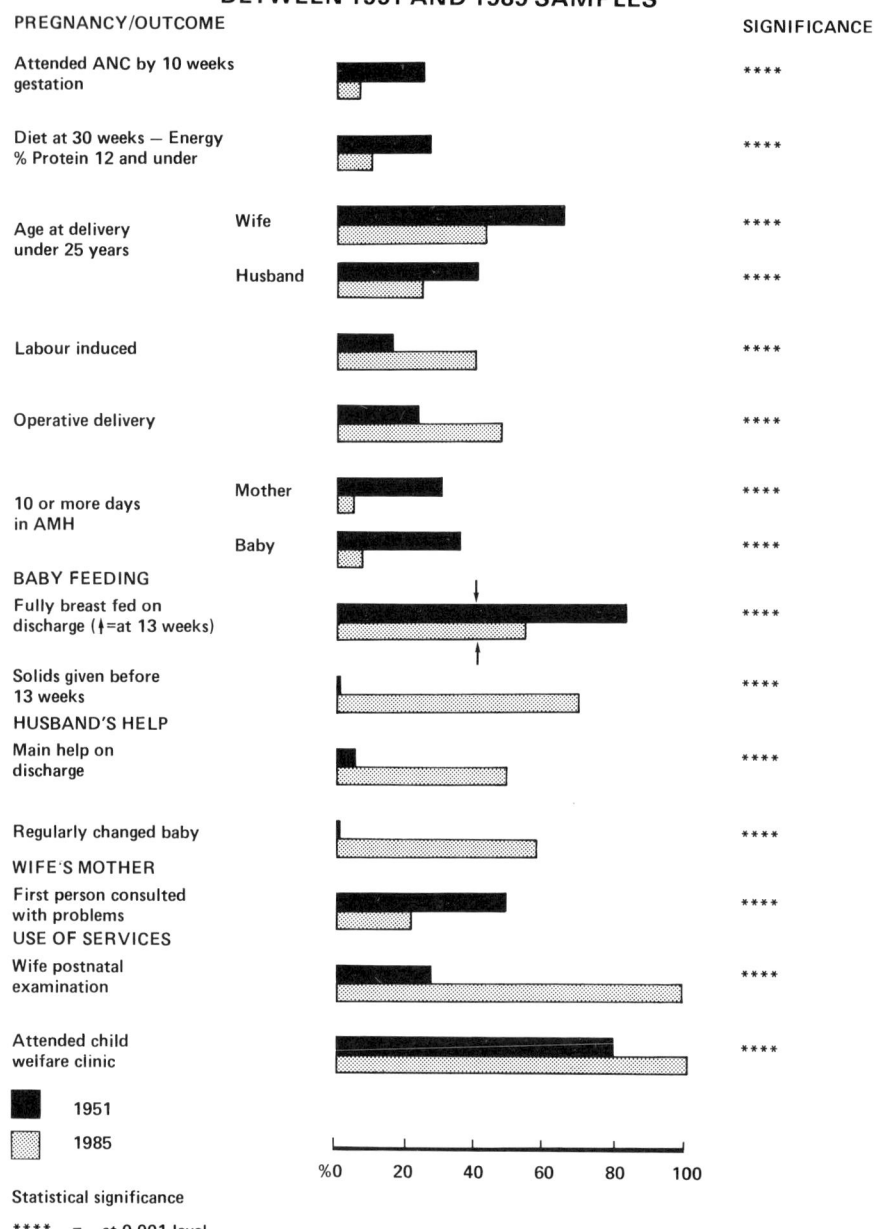

FIGURE 12.1 c SOME SIGNIFICANT STATISTICAL DIFFERENCES BETWEEN 1951 AND 1985 SAMPLES

PREGNANCY/OUTCOME

SIGNIFICANCE

Attended ANC by 10 weeks gestation — ****

Diet at 30 weeks — Energy % Protein 12 and under — ****

Age at delivery under 25 years — Wife **** — Husband ****

Labour induced — ****

Operative delivery — ****

10 or more days in AMH — Mother **** — Baby ****

BABY FEEDING

Fully breast fed on discharge (✝=at 13 weeks) — ****

Solids given before 13 weeks — ****

HUSBAND'S HELP

Main help on discharge — ****

Regularly changed baby — ****

WIFE'S MOTHER

First person consulted with problems — ****

USE OF SERVICES

Wife postnatal examination — ****

Attended child welfare clinic — ****

■ 1951

▨ 1985

%0 20 40 60 80 100

Statistical significance

**** = at 0.001 level

Some Experiences of the 1985 Postnatal Sample

This Appendix reports certain information only available for the 1985 postnatal sample of 150 women.

ANTENATAL CLASSES

When asked about their intention to attend the antenatal classes, five women said that they would not be going because they were either 'too busy' or it was 'too far to go' and none of these had attended (Table A.1). A further nine women were uncertain about going, but some of these did attend after they had had details of the classes from the Health Visitor. The vast majority said that they 'intended to go to the classes'.

Admission to AMH prevented a few women from going (Table A.1). Two women had withdrawn; they described the only class they had attended as 'a waste of time'. Overall 85% of the sample had attended most, if not all, the classes—17% dismissed the classes as 'useless' as a preparation for labour and delivery, 46% had derived 'some help' from them, and 22% had found them 'a great help'. The women had appreciated the tuition in breathing

TABLE A.1

EXPERIENCE WITH ANTENATAL CLASSES 1985 POSTNATAL SAMPLE ONLY

	Intention to attend			Total	
	Yes	Uncertain	No		
	No.	No.	No.	No.	%
Attended					
Very helpful	33	—	—	33	22
Some help	68	1	—	69	46
Useless	22	4	—	26	17
Discontinued					
Admitted AMH	7	—	—	7⎱	6
Other	1	1	—	2⎰	
Did not attend					
Admitted to AMH	1	—	1	2⎱	9
Other	4	3	4	11⎰	
Total	136	9	5	150	100

exercises and methods of relaxation, and reported that what they had learned at the classes had helped them to understand what was going on during labour and delivery. This particularly applied to women who ended up having a caesarean section or a forceps delivery, and helped to allay their fears and, therefore, to facilitate their co-operation. The opportunity to get to know other primigravidae had been important, particularly as the classes had been held at a time when some women were beginning to feel socially isolated after giving up work. Several valued the friendships which developed through attendance at the classes and had been maintained postnatally.

Five women had attended classes provided by the National Childbirth Trust, in addition to those provided through the clinic. These women had found the NCT classes particularly helpful, and were impressed by the training and experience of the instructors. Details of the husbands' attendance at antenatal classes were not routinely collected, although it was known that the majority intended to go. Only one woman did not wish her husband to be involved in what she considered to be 'women's business'.

LABOUR AND DELIVERY

At the thirteen weeks postnatal home visit, the women were asked for details of their labour and delivery for comparison with the hospital records (Table A.2) and also for comment on their experiences.

TABLE A.2

COMPARISON OF RECORDED AND REPORTED EXPERIENCES OF LABOUR
AND DELIVERY—1985 POSTNATAL SAMPLE OF 150 WOMEN

		Agreement	Recorded in medical notes but not reported	Reported by women but not recorded in medical notes
Induction	%	94	3	3
Method of delivery	%	100	—	—
Analgesic/anaesthetic				
Gas and air	%	73	3	24
Pethidine	%	92	6	2
Epidural	%	99	1	—
General anaesthetic	%	100	—	—
Other	%	59	38	3
Episiotomy	%	95	3	2
Perineal stitches	%	100	—	—
Complications				
APH	%	92	7	1
PE—mild	%	82	16	2
moderate/severe	%	96	4	—
Fetal distress	%	54	45	1

The women's statements and the medical records usually agreed on induction and the reasons for it. However, four women thought that they had been induced when according to the medical records an ARM or syntocin drip had been given to accelerate labour already under way. Conversely, four women said that labour had started spontaneously when it was recorded as being induced. Six of the sixty women who reported that labour had been induced, were unsure about the reason.

All women agreed with the recorded method of delivery and the majority could give the reason for an operative procedure. However, one woman who had a CS and one who had a forceps delivery were unwilling to discuss their experiences, while one woman maintained that she did not now why she had had a CS.

Rates of agreement between recorded and reported use of analgesics were variable (Table A.2). There was only a 73% agreement between recorded use of gas and air and what the women reported. The indications were that casual, intermittent or brief use was not recorded in the medical notes. Whereas thirty-six women said that they had used gas and air, but this was not recorded, five women did not report having used it contrary to the records. There was a much higher rate of agreement between the records and the womens' accounts in the use of pethidine, epidurals, general anaesthetic and other methods. Indeed, all women agreed with the records on whether or not they had had a general anaesthetic, and with one exception whether they had had an epidural. The exception was a woman who had requested an epidural, but labour had progressed to the second stage as it was being administered:—she thought the epidural had not been started, but the obstetric record contradicted this. Twelve women did not agree with the records on the use of pethidine, three said they had used it and nine did not mention it. Also three women did not report 'other' pain relief recorded as given a pudendal block, diamorphine and the pulsar respectively.

Initially, the women were not questioned in detail about their experiences in using the various methods of pain relief and the information is available for only about three-quarters of those who reported using each method. Overall the women were most satisfied with epidurals and least satisfied with pethidine (Table A.3). The majority of women who commented on their experience with an epidural were enthusiastic (61%) and spoke in superlatives such as 'super' and 'wonderful' or 'like a magic wand' and said they would want to have it again. An epidural had given 'some help' to another 24% of women. Those who had had a CS under an epidural had appreciated being conscious during the operation, and this had allowed their husbands to be present. However, four women complained that the epidural had not worked and three had experienced unpleasant side effects—two had had epidural taps and one had become hypotensive.

The majority of women had been dissatisfied with pethidine—45% said that it had been useless, while a further 18% complained of unpleasant side effects, mainly nausea and feelings of disorientation. One-fifth of the women said that pethidine had helped them to relax, but in some cases the effects had been very temporary and a second injection had given little relief. Only

TABLE A.3

WOMEN'S ASSESSMENT OF PAIN RELIEF AND BREATHING EXERCISES—
1985 POSTNATAL SAMPLE OF 150 WOMEN

	Gas and Air	Pethidene	Epidural	Breathing exercises
(n)	(85)	(76)	(46)	(69)
	%	%	%	%
Very helpful	31	15	61	33
Some help	16	22	24	56
Disliked	19	18	6	—
Useless	34	45	9	11
Total	100	100	100	100

one in seven of the women who commented on pethidine had found it very helpful, but they were guarded in their praise.

One half of the women who commented on their use of gas and air were dissatisfied (Table A.3). Most of these said it had been useless, sometimes because they had found it difficult to co-ordinate the timing of use with contractions as labour progressed. Feelings of nausea and disorientation had upset some women. In contrast some of the women who had found gas and air a considerable help in relieving the pain had enjoyed the 'woozy' feeling which others had detested. As a distraction, attempts to use gas and air had given some help to 18% of the women.

The few women who had used the pulsar were enthusiastic about it. The three who had been given chlormethiazole (a rapid acting anticonvulsant) said that they had no recollection of their labour.

Antenatally, women are encouraged to do breathing exercises and advised how these can help during labour. The medical records do not record whether women use breathing exercises, but about half the women reported trying to put into practice what they had learnt at the antenatal classes. The majority had found breathing exercises 'very helpful' (33%) or 'some help' (39%). In the early stages of labour breathing exercises had been appreciated as 'a helpful diversion' or as 'something to do', but as labour had progressed the exercises had been abandoned as the pain became too severe or the women had run out of energy. A few women dismissed such exercises as useless, explaining that they had felt too anxious to put them into practice. It was exceptional for women to rely solely on breathing exercises to help them through labour.

Macintrye (1981) reports verbatim comments by Aberdeen primigravidae on their varied experiences with different methods of pain relief and anaesthesia.

The women and medical records agreed on whether there had been perineal stitching, but eight women disagreed with the medical notes on whether they had had an episiotomy (Table A.2). Three women reported having an episiotomy in contradiction to the medical records, while five women did not report such intervention.

Whether or not they had antepartum haemorrhage was accurately reported by most women. However, eight of the twenty-three women for whom it was recorded did not report it and two were unsure. One woman thought that she had bled before labour started in contrast to what was recorded. At times it can be difficult even for obstetricians to differentiate between APH and 'a show' at the onset of labour.

The significance of a raised blood pressure and the diagnosis of PE was sometimes confused. Six women recorded as having moderate PE did not report this. One woman admitted to the antenatal ward for several weeks on account of PE said that she had felt very well and could not understand the concern and 'what all the fuss was about' until she saw an episode of *Dallas* on television some weeks later in which one of the stars was in hospital with a similar condition. It was only after this that she realised the potential seriousness of PE and appreciated the care and attention given to her at AMH. Over half the women recorded as having hypertension or mild PE never mentioned it. In contrast a few others said that they had had a raised blood pressure, but presumably it had not been high enough or sustained long enough to be classified as hypertension. Although most babies were recorded as distressed during labour, it was evident that in most cases this gave no cause for alarm and the diagnosis was not communicated to the mothers. One woman's statement that her baby had been distressed was unsubstantiated.

In general, women reported their obstetric experience as recorded in the medical notes. Differences were usually easily explicable in terms of the strict coding criteria applied by obstetricians.

Nearly all the husbands were said to have been keen to share the experience of childbirth (Table A.4) and were encouraged by their wives to

TABLE A.4

HUSBAND'S PRESENCE AT LABOUR AND DELIVERY BY INTENTION—1985
POSTNATAL SAMPLE ONLY

| Present at | Intention to be present | | | Total | |
| | Yes | Uncertain | No | | |
	No.	No.	No.	No.	%
Labour and delivery	122	6	1	129	86
Labour only	8[6]	—	3	11[6]	7
Delivery only	3	—	—	3	2
Neither	3[3]	3	1[1]	7[4]	5
Total No.	136[9]	9	5[1]	150[10]	
%	91	6	3		100

( ) CS under general anaesthetic

be present. At the time of the antenatal interview, nine wives were unsure whether their husbands would be present mostly because of work commitments, e.g. they were due to be offshore about the time the baby was due. Five wives said that their husbands definitely did not intend to be present in the Labour Ward because they were 'too squeamish', scared of hospitals or 'too much of a coward'. Only two women did not wish their husbands to be present at the birth—in addition to the one referred to earlier who viewed it as 'women's business'—another was not getting on well with her husband, but later they were reconciled and he did attend.

In the event, 86% of the wives, including those who had a CS under an epidural anaesthetic, had their husbands with them throughout labour and delivery. Six of the nine men whose attendance had originally been uncertain did manage to be present, usually after rearranging work schedules; and one man who totally changed his mind about being present was reported to have found it a most rewarding experience.

Eleven men were present during labour, but not at the delivery. Eight had always hoped to be present, but six of them were sent away while their wives had a CS under general anaesthetic; this was anticipated for another woman who was removed to the theatre, but ended up having a forceps delivery. The eighth man felt overwhelmed and near to fainting, so voluntarily withdrew rather than see his wife have an episiotomy and forceps delivery. Of three men who had not wished to be present, two visited their wives intermittently during labour only, while the third, who had changed his mind, was sent away when forceps were required.

Three men who had intended to be present throughout had to be called from their work and arrived only just in time for the delivery.

Only seven of the 150 women did not have their husbands present at some time during labour and delivery, and four of these had a CS under general anaesthetic from which husbands are normally excluded. Three husbands had intended to be be present, but one of the wives was admitted for an elective CS and the other two were transferred to the theatre very soon after admission. The only woman who always wished to exclude her husband eventually had a CS under general anaesthetic, and so he would not have been present at the delivery in any case.

Three men who had been uncertain about attending were not present at the delivery. Discretion prevailed in the case of one husband who stayed away for health reasons. Work prevented two other men from being with their wives as one was away from Aberdeen while the owner of a business could not get away in time.

In general, the women were full of praise for the way their husbands had been welcomed in the Labour Ward and made to feel an integral part of the procedure. The few complaints were usually attributed to the staff being so busy, e.g. one husband had been distressed 'at being forgotten' when his wife, who was taken away for a CS under general anaesthetic, in fact had a forceps delivery at which he could have been present. It was not always understood why husbands were asked to leave if their wives had a general anaesthetic. Although they might not have elected to remain, they would have liked to be given the choice. After being present during a long labour the husbands sometimes 'felt cheated'. As one woman said, 'If he felt able to stay then I would have liked him to be present.'

The women described the feeling of security that having their husbands there had given them as they had never been left alone during labour. Apprehension about how the husbands would behave in the situation was usually allayed as the husbands became 'fascinated' by what was going on in the Labour Ward and became interested in, although sometimes alarmed by, the technology. Many husbands were said to have been surprised if not appalled at what their wives had to go through, but feelings of helplessness had been partially relieved by taking an active part in assisting their wives with breathing exercises, or back rubbing, or by acting as a physical support, which occasionally left them with painful bruises. No husband had fainted although one came near to it and a few others were said to be nearing the end of their endurance, but glad that they 'had managed to survive' as witnessing the birth had been 'great'.

Whatever the experience the great majority of wives reported that their husbands 'wouldn't have missed it for anything'—a few having forfeited wages to be present.

Reaction to total experience. The women were asked to try and categorise their own and their husbands' feelings about their total experience of childbirth (Table A.5). Although these ranged from the euphoric to the traumatic, most used expressions such as 'enjoyable', 'alright' or indicated that the experience had been 'off putting' and these were the categories used for analysis. About one-fifth of wives and half the husbands were said to have found the experience 'enjoyable'. The wives were more likely to

TABLE A.5

WIFE'S REACTION TO TOTAL EXPERIENCE BY HUSBAND'S REACTION— 1985 POSTNATAL SAMPLE ONLY

Husband's reaction	Wife's reaction				Total	
	Enjoyed	Alright	Off-putting	Other		
					No.	%
Enjoyed	29	25	9	9	72	51
Alright	1	27	4	6	38	27
Off-putting	—	4	8	—	12	8
Other	2	8	2	8	20	14
No comment	—	2	2	4	8*	—
Total No.	32	66	25	27	150	
%	21	44	17	18		100

Wife v Husband $\lambda^2_{(3)} = 28.3353$ $p \leqslant 0.001$

* Seven did not attend AMH
  One intermittently present during labour only

consider it as 'alright'. About one-in-seven women, however, had found it 'off putting': twice as many wives as husbands. The feelings of some wives and husbands could only be described as 'other'. Typically they were very mixed, reactions being different to different parts of the experience, e.g. enjoying the early stage of labour, finding the epidural 'off putting' and the birth a 'non-event'.

The reactions to their total experiences were very varied and specific to the individual women and their husbands. What one person enjoyed another found off putting, largely depending on what they had expected or wanted. For example, one woman was delighted to end up having a CS which she had always wanted, while another found this greatly distressing because having been deprived of the experience 'of giving birth' she felt it was 'all a bit weird' and found it difficult to accept that the baby was hers. Whereas one described an epidural as 'murder', another said it was 'marvellous'.

Numbers are small, but indicate that for both the wives and the husbands enjoyment was inversely associated with the use of analgesics and anaesthetics (and by implication with longer labours) and with operative delivery; PE also adversely affected the women's reactions whereas APH, episiotomy and perineal stitches seemed to have had less impact (Table A.6).

Overall 20% of the couples who had shared all or part of the experience had enjoyed the birth of their first child whilst 6% had found it off putting, though not necessarily sufficiently so to deter them from having another. The majority of couples, however, were reported to have viewed the experiences rather differently from one another (Table A.5).

The following examples picked at random, two from each sub-category, illustrate the similarities and the differences in the couples' experiences.

TABLE A.6

PERCENTAGE IN EACH EXPERIENCE CATEGORY BY METHOD OF DELIVERY, COMPLICATIONS AND PAIN RELIEF—1985 POSTNATAL SAMPLE

	Wife			Husband*		
	Enjoyed	Alright	Off-putting	Enjoyed	Alright	Off-putting
(n)	(32)	(66)	(25)	(72)	(38)	(12)
Operative delivery	31	48	56	36	55	50
Episiotomy	59	62	52	62	65	25
Stitches	75	79	72	79	81	42
APH	12	16	12	11	18	25
Hypertension/PE	34	41	44	43	47	25
Gas and air	44	56	60	54	53	75
Pethidine	53	63	84	67	53	83
Epidural	31	41	68	40	45	58
General anaesthetic	3	4	16	3	8	25

* Excluding no comment

1. Similar category for wife and husband

(a)'*Enjoyed*'

    (i)   Experience 'wonderful' for wife, 'fantastic' for husband; a short, straight-forward labour with minimum use of gas and air ending in a spontaneous delivery, described as 'a very positive experience for us both'.

    (ii)   A 'tremendous' experience although tiring until given an epidural—the spontaneous birth was 'exhilarating'; husband felt welcomed and involved.

(b)'*Alright*'

    (i)   Both disappointed because a long labour ended in a CS under a general anaesthetic; neither had found the experience pleasurable, but it had not deterred them from wanting another child.

    (ii)   Wife became distressed towards the end of a long, slow labour and had a forceps delivery; husband found it rather tedious, but was unhappy about the intervention. Both were glad they had shared the experience.

(c)'*Off putting*'

    (i)   Both distressed because a long labout had ended in a CS on account of fetal distress. They would only contemplate having another baby if the wife could be guaranteed an elective CS.

    (ii)   Labour had been 'awful', nothing had helped and the epidural had been given 'too late', prior to a spontaneous delivery. The experience had been traumatic to both and only served to reinforce their intention only to have one child. The wife said she would like to be sterilised.

(d)'*Other*'

    (i)   They had enjoyed the early stage of labour; the epidural was 'terrible because it did not work', and the wife ended up having a forceps delivery. The husband was very distressed at the outcome. Both had nightmares for quite a long time afterwards.

    (ii)   Both enjoyed it until the baby turned during labour; afterwards it was very painful, and the husband had been upset to see his wife in such a state. An epidural worked well, but the husband was distressed by the forceps delivery.

2. Different category for wife and husband

(a) *Wife 'enjoyed'*

    (i)   'Alright' for husband who became squeamish at the time of (spontaneous) delivery.

    (ii)   'Other' for husband who found it difficult to see his wife suffering, but was glad he stayed because the spontaneous birth was 'wonderful'.

(b) *Wife 'alright'*

    (i)   'Off putting' for husband who found it an ordeal and was badly bruised by wife. He had said that he would not have believed what she had to go through if he had not seen it for himself. She had found it all 'worth it, but not enjoyable' (spontaneous delivery).

    (ii)   'Other' for husband who claimed it was 'an experience'. He had accepted being there as a challenge because he did not like the sight of blood and felt quite triumphant, but was relieved that his wife had had a short labour and spontaneous delivery.

(c) *Wife 'off putting'*

    (i)   'Enjoyed' by husband. 'Murder' was how this wife described her experience—PE, and forceps delivery under epidural, whereas to the husband it was a short, painless labour and seeing the baby born was 'terrific'.

    (ii)   'Other' for husband. Everything had gone well until an epidural 'ended in disaster' and the wife had a dural tap, so that the husband's optimistic enthusiasm soon turned to anxiety about his wife and the baby (forceps).

(d) *Wife 'other'*

    (i)   Husband 'enjoyed'. The wife had found it initially exciting, but quickly became very tired and had very vague memories of the birth because of the effects of pethidine, whereas the husband had been 'totally fascinated' by the whole procedure and enjoyed it (spontaneous delivery).

    (ii)   'Alright' for husband. 'Nerve-racking' was how the wife explained her reaction, as she felt confused and became very worried about the baby when forceps were used. Although the husband felt involved and was able to help he was too anxious about his wife to really enjoy it.

No type of labour or delivery guaranteed that the couple would find it a pleasurable experience. It depended on what they expected and on whether the assistance and the outcome were what they wanted. Whether the experience was likely to be more pleasurable because less intervention was required, or whether less intervention was required because the couple were enjoying the experience and had a more positive attitude to childbirth, is not determined. Long labour and complications requiring intervention and operative delivery were certainly exacting and sometimes daunting experiences for couples. Within each category of respone, some womn talked of the importance of the shared experience in their partnership and in generating a family feeling.

BIRTHWEIGHT

The women were asked their baby's birthweight, and their reports were compared with the hospital records. At AMH the weight is recorded to the nearest 10g, but with very few exceptions the women reported the weight in pounds and ounces and this had to be converted to grammes. Thus some slight discrepancies might be expected and the woman's report has been taken to agree if the converted weight was within 10g of that recorded in AMH. Overall 76% of the women reported their baby's birthweight as that recorded in the medical records and a further 17% gave it to within 1oz. Only four women were 50g or more out, the largest discrepancy being an under-reporting of 144g (about 5ozs).

SMOKING

At the thirteen weeks postnatal visit, thirty-nine primiparae (26%) said that they smoked—fourteen women smoked less than ten cigarettes daily, eight smoked ten to nineteen a day and sixteen smoked twenty or more. Over half these women (54%) said that they had cut down their smoking after they became pregnant, whereas 13% said that they had smoked more, particularly in the later stage of pregnancy after they had stopped work and had time on their hands, or were beginning to feel apprehensive about their confinement.

Two women who said that they had given up smoking by the thirty week antenatal interview were smoking again by thirteen weeks postnatally. One blamed AMH for not prohibiting smoking in the dayroom—with others around her smoking she disliked being a passive smoker and started smoking again. (More recently, restrictions on smoking in AMH have been increased.)

The indications were that, in the long term, pregnancy made little difference to the smoking habits of these particular primiparae, unless some specific health problem had intervened. For example, one woman described how she had cut down her smoking during pregnancy, but postnatally was soon smoking her usual 10-15 cigarettes a day. Another much heavier smoker who was not enjoying motherhood and was finding 'life boring' at thirteen weeks, said that it was smoking that 'kept her sane'. Graham (1976; 1984) in studies of health and the family reported on the way in which some women find that smoking relieves unbearable tension and helps them to be more responsible mothers. A woman whose high blood pressure caused concern and who had this monitored for several weeks postnatally was sufficiently alarmed to have given up smoking; she said that she had only smoked one cigarette since the birth.

SEXUAL INTERCOURSE POSTNATALLY

In an attempt to discover how childbirth had affected sex, the women were asked how soon after the birth they had resumed intercourse and if they had encountered any difficulties. Seven of the 150 women said that they were still abstaining because of slow healing vaginal wounds, continued bleeding, tender abdominal scar or excessive tiredness and loss of interest. Most of these, however, were already taking the pill, in two cases in the hope that bleeding would be reduced.

On average, couples resumed intercourse around 5.4 weeks, about the time of the wife's postnatal examination. Some women had preferred to wait until after this in order 'to be sure that everything was all right'. However, 28% said that they had resumed within a month of the birth and 11% had waited over two months. The timing depended on many factors, such as how quickly stitches and wounds healed, bleeding stopped or tenderness from abdominal scars diminished. In some cases, where the husband worked away from home some of the time, the timing had been partially dictated by his pattern of work. One-fifth of the women (20%) reported some problems initially, mainly pain and tenderness, and at thirteen weeks postnatally, eleven women (7%) complained that they still found intercourse painful or very uncomfortable.

Four women said that they had lost interest in having intercourse and one of these had not had sex since the birth. They tended to blame their excessive tiredness, but one thought that her nightmarish experience in having a forceps delivery had put her off sex. One woman voiced what many others seemed to feel when she said 'sex has moved down my list of priorities'.

References

Adams, E M and Finlayson A (1961), 'Familial aspects of pre-eclampsia and hypertension in pregnancy', *Lancet*, ii: 1373–5.

Aitken-Swan, J and Baird, D (1965), 'Circumcision and cancer of the cervix', *British Journal of Cancer*, 19: 217–27.

Aitken-Swan, J and Baird, D (1966), Cancer of the uterine cervix in Aberdeenshire. Parts I and II, *British Journal of Cancer*, 22: 624–41.

Baird, D (1945), 'The influence of social and economic factors on stillbirths and neonatal deaths', *Journal of Obstetrics and Gynaecology of British Empire*, 52: 339–66.

——(1946), 'Variations in reproductive pattern according to social class', *Lancet*, ii: 41–4.

——(1947), 'Social class and fetal mortality', *Lancet*, ii: 531–5.

——(1948), 'Nutrition in pregnancy', *Practitioner*, 160: 34–40.

——(1949), 'Social factors in obstetrics', *Lancet*, i: 1079–83.

——(1952), 'The causes and prevention of difficult labour', *American Journal of Obstetrics and Gynecology*, 63: 1200–12.

——(1955), 'Caesarean section—its use in difficult labour in primigravidae', *British Medical Journal*, 2: 1159–63.

——(1963), 'The contribution of operative obstetrics to the prevention of perinatal death', *Journal of Obstetrics and Gynaecology of British Commonwealth*, 70: 204–18.

——(1965), 'A Fifth Freedom?', *British Medical Journal*, 2: 1141–8.

——(1969), 'Perinatal mortality', *Lancet*, i: 511–15.

——(1971), 'The obstetrician and society', *Journal of Biosocial Science,* Suppl. 3, 91–111.

——(1985), 'Changing problems and priorities in obstetrics', *British Journal of Obstetrics and Gynaecology*, 92: 115–21.

Baird, D and Illsley, R (1953) 'Environment and childbearing', *Proceedings of the Royal Society of Medicine*, 46, 2: 53–9.

Baird, D, Thomson, A M and Duncan, E H L (1953), 'The causes and prevention of stillbirths and first week deaths', Part II. Evidence from clinical records. *Journal of Obstetrics and Gynaecology of British Empire*, 60: 17–30.

Baird, D, Walker, J and Thomson, A M (1954), 'The causes and prevention of stillbirths and first week deaths', Part III. A classification of deaths by clinical causes. *Journal of Obstetrics and Gynaecology of British Empire*, 61: 433–48.

Baird, D, Anderson, A R M and Turnbull, A C (1968), 'Influence of induction of labour on the caesarean section rates, duration of labour and perinatal mortality in Aberdeen primigravidae 1938–1966', *Journal of Obstetrics and Gynaecology of British Commonwealth*, 75: 800–11.

Balfour, M (1938), 'The effect of occupation on pregnancy and neonatal mortality', *Public Health Journal of Society of Medical Officers of Health*, 51: 106–11.

Bernard, R M (1952), 'The size and shape of the female pelvis', *Edinburgh Medical Journal*, 59: 1–16.

Billewicz, W Z, (1972), 'A note on birthweight correlation in full siblings', *Journal of Biosocial Science*, 4: 455–60.

Birch, H, Richardson, S A, Baird, D, Illsley, R and Horobin, G W (1970), *Mental subnormality in a community: a clinical and epidemiological study* (Williams and Wilkins Co., Baltimore).

Blaxter, M (1980), *The health of the children: a review of research on the place of health in cycles of disadvantage* (Heinemann Educational Books, London).

Blaxter, M and Paterson, E (1982), *Mothers and daughters* (Heinemann Educational Books, London).

Bone, M (1980), 'Trends in contraceptive practice among married couples', *Health Trends*, 12: 87–90.

Bonney, N L (1986), 'Social and economic change in Aberdeen 1971–1981'. Report prepared for the Economic and Social Research Council.

Brown, A and Kiernan, K E (1981), 'Cohabitation in Great Britain: evidence from the General Household Survey', *Population Trends*, 25: 4–10 (HMSO).

Butler, N R and Alberman, E D (eds) (1969), *Perinatal problems* (E and S Livingstone, Edinburgh).

Butler, N R and Bonham, D G (1963), *Perinatal mortality* (E and S Livingstone, Edinburgh).

Campbell, D M and Samphier, M (1988), 'Birthweight standards for twins'. In: *Twinning and Twins* (eds) MacGillivray, I, Campbell, D M and Thompson, B (John Wiley, Chichester).

Campbell, D M, Campbell-Brown, B M, Jandial, L and MacGillivray, I (1979), 'Maternal energy intake in pregnancy and its relation to maternal fetal factors', *Proceedings of the Nutrition Society*, 38: 53A.

Campbell, D M, Campbell-Brown, B M, Jandial, L and MacGillivray, I (1982), 'Maternal energy intake in pregnancy and its relation to maternal fetal factors', *Proceedings of the Nutrition Society*, 41: 30A.

Carr-Hill, R and Pritchard, C (1985), *The development and exploitation of empirical birthweight standards* (Macmillan Press Ltd, London).

Carr-Hill, R, Campbell, D M, Hall, M H and Meredith, A (1987), 'Is birthweight determined genetically?' *British Medical Journal*, 295: 687–90.

Cartwright, A (1978), 'Recent trends in family building and contraception', *Studies on Medical Population Subjects*. No. 34 (HMSO, London).

Central Statistical Office (1985). Social Trends, 15 (HMSO, London).

Chamberlain, G (ed) (1984), *Pregnant women at work* (Royal Society of Medicine and Macmillan Press, London).

Chng, P, Hall, M and MacGillivray, I (1980), 'An audit of antenatal care: the value of the first antenatal visit'. *British Medical Journal*, 281: 1184–6.

Cleary, J and Sheppherdson, B (1981a), 'The presentation of motherhood'. Report on motherhood in Swansea: a study of the sources of information used by first-time mothers. Department of Sociology and Anthropology, University College of Swansea.

Cleary, J and Sheppherdson, B (1981b), 'The Fyynone fathers'. Motherhood in Swansea—Suppl. Paper 2. Medical Sociology Research Centre, University College of Swansea.

Committee on Medical Aspects of Food Policy (1980). Present day practice in infant feeding. Report of a working party of the Panel on Child Nutrition Committee on medical aspects of Food Policy. (HMSO, London).

Crammond, W A (1954), 'Psychological aspects of uterine dysfunction', *Lancet*, ii: 1241–5.

Department of Health and Social Security (1979). Report on Health and Social Studies, No. 15. Recommended daily amounts of food energy and nutrients of groups of people in the UK (HMSO, London).

Department of Health and Social Security (1980). Inequalities in health. Report of a research working group chaired by Sir Douglas Black (HMSO, London).

Douglas, J W B (1948), *Maternity in Great Britain* (Oxford University Press, London).

Duncan, E H L, Baird, D and Thomson, A M (1952), 'The causes and prevention of stillbirths and first week deaths'. Part I. The evidence of vital statistics. *Journal of Obstetrics and Gynaecology of British Empire*, 59: 183–95.

Edwards, H and Thompson, B (1971), 'Who are the fatherless?' *New Society*, No 436: 192–3.

Firth, R and Djamour, J (1956), 'Kinship in South Borough'. In: *Two Studies of Kinship in London* (ed) Firth, R. (University of London, Athlone Press).

Fraser, C M (1983), 'Selected perinatal procedures: scientific basis for use and psychosocial effects', *Acta Obstetricia et Gynecologica Scandinavica*, Suppl. 117.

Fraser, C M (1984), 'The follow-up study: psychological aspects'. In *Low birthweight: a medical, psychological and social study* (eds) Illsley, R and Mitchell, R G (John Wiley, Chichester).

Fraser, C M (1987) Personal communication.

Fullerton, W T (1973). Report of a working party on contraception in the North-East of Scotland. Unpublished.

General Register Office (1950). *Classification of occupations* (HMSO, London).

General Register Office Edinburgh (1953). Census 1951: City of Aberdeen Report on the 15th Census of Scotland, Vol. 1, Part 3 (HMSO, Edinburgh).

Gill, D G, Reid, G D B and Smith, D M (1971), 'Sex education, press and parental perceptions', *Health Education Journal*, 30: 2.

Graham, H (1976), 'Smoking in pregnancy: the attitude of expectant mothers', Social Science and Medicine, 10: 399–405.

——(1979), 'Prevention of health: every mother's business'. In: *The Society and the Family*, Harris, C C (ed), *Sociological Review Monograph*, No 28: 160–85.

——(1984), *Women, health and the family* (Wheatsheaf Books, Brighton).

Hall, M, Chng, P and MacGillivray, I (1980), 'Is routine antental care worthwhile?' *Lancet*, ii: 78–80.

Hall, M, Macintyre, S and Porter, M (1985), *Antenatal care assessed: a case study of innovation in Aberdeen* (Aberdeen University Press).

Health Education Council (1987). The health divide: inequalities in health in the 1980s. A review prepared by Margaret Whitehead.

Hope, E, Marr, J, Stevenson, J and Thomson, A M (1956). The food habits of pregnant women in Aberdeen. Quoted by Illsley, R (1956a).

Hytten, F E (1954), 'Clinical and chemical studies in human lactation'. Parts 1-9. *British Medical Journal*, i: 175–82; 249–55; 912–15; 1410–13. ii: 844–5; 1447–52.

——(1984), 'The effect of work on placental function and fetal growth'. In: *Pregnant women at work,* (ed) Chamberlain, G (Royal Society of Medicine and Macmillan Press, London).

Hytten, F E and Leitch, I (1971), *The physiology of human pregnancy,* 2nd edn (Blackwell Scientific Press, Oxford).

Hytten, F E and MacQueen, I A G (1954), 'Artificial feeding and energy requirements of young infants', *Lancet*, ii: 836–9.

Illsley, R (1955), 'Social class and selection and class, differences in relation to stillbirths and infant deaths, *British Medical Journal*, ii: 1520–4.

——(1956a), 'The social background to first pregnancy'. Unpublished PhD Thesis, University of Aberdeen.

——(1956b), 'The duration of antenatal care', *Medical Officer*, 96: 107–11.

——(1980), *Professional or public health: sociology in health and medicine* (Nuffield Provincial Hospital Trust, London).

Illsley, R and Mitchell, R G (eds) (1984), *Low birthweight: a medical, psychological and social study* (John Wiley, Chichester).

Illsley, R and Thompson, B (1961), 'Women from broken homes', *Sociological Review*, 9, No. 1: 27–54.

Illsley, R and Thompson, B (1976) 'Social characteristics identifying women at risk for premature delivery'. In: *Prevention of handicap through antenatal care* (eds) Turnbull, A C and Woodford, FP (Associated Scientific Publications, Amsterdam).

Illsley, R, Billewicz, W Z and Thomson, A M (1954), 'Prematurity and paid work during pregnancy', *British Journal of Preventive and Social Medicine*, 8: 153–6.

Illsley, R, Finlayson, A and Thompson, B (1963), 'The motivation and characteristics of internal migrants', Parts I and II. *Millbank Memorial Fund Quarterly*, 41, 2: 115–43; 3: 217–48.

Ingelman-Sundberg, A (1958), 'The value of antenatal massage of nipples and expression of colostrum', *Journal of Obstetrics and Gynaecology of British Empire*, 65: 448–9.

Jackson, B (1984), *Fatherhood* (Allen and Unwin, London).

Johnstone, F D, Campbell-Brown, M, Campbell, D M and MacGillivray, I (1981), 'Measurement of variables—quality control', *American Journal of Clinical Nutrition*, 34: 804–6.

Knight, I (1984), *The height and weight of adults in Great Britain* (OPCS, HMSO, London).

Lancet, Leading Article (1966), 'Father in the labour ward', *Lancet*, i: 699.

Lancet, Leading Article (1986), 'Should third stage of labour be managed actively?', *Lancet*, ii: 22–4.

Lowell, J P and Mackie, J R (1983), 'Computerised dietary calculations: interactive approach updated'. In: Human Nutrition: Applied Nutrition, 37A: 36–40.

McCance, R A and Widdowson, E M (1946), Special report of the General Medical Research Council, No 235, 2nd edn. London.

Macfarlane, A and Mugford, M (1984), *Birth counts: statistics of pregnancy and childbirth*. National Perinatal Epidemiology Unit in collaboration with OPCS, (HMSO, London).

Macgregor, J E and Baird, D (1963), 'Detection of cervical carcinoma in the general population', *British Medical Journal*, i: 1631–6.

McIntosh, J (1985). A consumer perspective on the health visiting service. Social Paediatric and Obstetric Research Unit, Glasgow.

Macintyre, S (1978), 'Obstetric routines in antenatal care'. In: *Relations between doctors and patients* (ed) Davis, A (Saxon House, London).

——(1981), 'Expectations and experiences of first pregnancy', MRC Medical Sociology Unit Occasional Paper No 5.

MacKee, L (1980), 'Fathers and childbirth', *The Health Visitor*, 53.

McKinlay, J B (1970), 'The new late comers for antenatal care', *British Journal of Preventive and Social Medicine*, 24, 1: 52–7.

MacQueen, I A G (1953). Report of the Medical Officer of Health for the City of Aberdeen for year 1952.

Mamelle, H and Laumon, B (1984), 'Occupational fatigue and preterm birth'. In: *Pregnant women at work* (ed) Chamberlain, G (Royal Society of Medicine and Macmillan Press, London).

Marr, J W, Hope, E B, Stevenson, J B and Thomson, A M (1955), 'Consumption of milk and vitamin concentrates by pregnant women in Aberdeen', *Proceedings of Nutrition Society*, 14: 7.

Martin, J and Roberts, C (1984), 'Women and employment: a lifetime perspective' (HMSO, London).

Maternity Alliance (1981). Pregnant at Work. A checklist for employers, personnel officers and trade union representatives.

Medical Research Council (1945). Accessory Food Factors Committee Report. Nutritive value of wartime foods. MRC (War) Memorandum, No 14.

Ministry of Agriculture, Food and Fisheries (1986). Household food consumption and expenditure 1984 (HMSO, London).

Ministry of Food (1950). Bulletin No 579, 3–10.

Ministry of Food (1954). Domestic food consumption and expenditure 1952: Annual Report of the National Food Survey Committee (HMSO, London).

National Advisory Committee on Nutrition Education (1983). A discussion paper on proposals for nutritional guidelines for health education in Britain. Health Education Council, London.

Nelson, T R (1955), A clinical study of pre-eclampsia. Parts I and II. *Journal of Obstetrics and Gynaecology of British Empire*, 62: 48–57; 58–66.

Oakley, A (1979), *Becoming a mother* (Martin Robertson, Oxford).

——(1980), *Women confined: towards a sociology of childbirth* (Martin Robertson, Oxford).

Office of Population Censuses and Surveys. Abortion statistics for England and Wales 1974–85. Annual Reports (HMSO, London).

Office of Population Censuses and Surveys. Birth statistics for England and Wales 1974–85. Annual Reports (HMSO, London).

Office of Population Censuses and Surveys (1980). Classification of occupations (HMSO, London).

Office of Population Censuses and Surveys (1985). Measuring socio-demographic change. Occasional Paper No 34.

Office of Population Censuses and Surveys, (1986). Mortality statistics, perinatal and infant: social and biological factors for 1984, Series DH3 No 17 (HMSO, London).

Ounsted, M, Scott, A and Moar, V A (1988), 'Constrained and unconstrained fetal growth: associations with some biological and pathological factors', *Annals of Human Biology*, 15: 2, 119–29.

Paul, A A and Southgate, D A T (1978), *McCance and Widdowson's Composition of Foods*, 4th edn (HMSO, London).

Payne, J (1975), 'Oil and housing in Aberdeen', *Health and Social Service Journal*, 85: 1798–9.

Prentice, A and Prentice A (1988), 'Reproduction against the odds', *New Scientist*, 1608.

Pritchard, C and Thompson, B (1982), 'Starting a family in Aberdeen 1961–79: the significance of illegitimacy and abortion', *Journal of Biosocial Science*, 14: 127–39.

Registrar General Scotland. Annual Reports 1950–85 (HMSO, Edinburgh).

Registrar General Scotland (1982). Census 1981 Reports for Grampian, Vol 1 (HMSO, Edinburgh).

Registrar General's Statistical Review of England and Wales. 1950–73. Annual Reports (HMSO, Edinburgh).

Richards, M and Bernal, J (1972), 'Effects of obstetric medication on mother-infant interaction and infant development'. In: *Psychosomatic medicine in Obstetrics and Gynaecology* (ed) Morris, N (Karger, Basle).

Richman, J and Goldthorp, W C (1978), 'Fatherhood: the social construction of pregnancy and birth'. In: *Place of Birth* (eds) Kitzinger, S and Davis, J A (Oxford University Press), pp 157–73.

Robson, E B (1955), 'Birthweight in cousins', *Annals of Human Genetics*, 19: 262–8.

Rowntree, G (1954), 'The finances of founding a family', *Scottish Journal of Political Economy*, 1: 201–32.

Samphier, M and Cunningham-Burley, S (1987). Personal communication.

Samphier, M and Thompson, B (1981), 'The Aberdeen Maternity and Neonatal Data Bank', In: *Prospective Longitudinal Research* (eds) Mednick, S A and Baert, A E (Oxford University Press).

Scott, E M (1954), 'A psychological enquiry amongst primigravidae: the role of psychological factors in childbearing, showing the relationship between intelligence, personality adjustment and maternal adjustment'. Unpublished PhD Thesis (University of Edinburgh).

Scott, E M and Thomson, A M (1956a), 'A psychological investigation of primigravidae'. Part I. Methods. *Journal of Obstetrics and Gynaecology of Britsh Empire*, 63: 331–7.

Scott, E M and Thomson, A M (1956b), 'A psychological investigation of primigravidae'. Part IV. Psychological factors and the clinical phenomena of labour. *Journal of Obstetrics and Gynaecology of Britsh Empire*, 63: 502–8.

Scott, E M, Illsley, R and Thomson, A M (1956a), 'A psychological investigation of primigravidae'. Part II. Maternal social class, age, physique and intelligence. *Journal of Obstetrics and Gynaecology of British Empire*, 63: 338–43.

Scott, E M, Illsley, R and Biles, E M (1956b), 'A psychological investigation of primigravidae'. Part III. Some aspects of maternal behaviour. *Journal of Obstetrics and Gynaecology of British Empire*, 63: 494–501.

Scottish Health Service. Scottish Health Statistics Annual Reports 1974–85 (HMSO, Edinburgh).

Spock, B (1958/1979), *Baby and child care*, 2nd and 4th edns (Bodley Head, London).

Stewart, D B and Scott, E M (1953), 'The assessment of efficiency in labour. Psychological factors related to labour', *Edinburgh Medical Journal*, 60: 49–58.

Sutherland, A I (1980), 'Genetic and non-genetic aspects of reproductive performance in man and the rabbit'. Unpublished PhD Thesis, University of Edinburgh.

Templeton, A A (1986) 'Human reproductive success', *Aberdeen Postgraduate Medical Bulletin*, 22: 1–7.

Thompson, B (1954), 'The housing of growing families in Aberdeen', *Medical Officer*, 91: 235–9.

——(1956), 'Social study of illegitimate maternities', *British Journal of Preventive and Social Medicine*, 10: 75–87.

——(1977), 'Problems of abortion in Britain—Aberdeen: a case study', *Population Studies*, 31: 143–54.

Thompson, B and Aitken-Swan, J (1973), 'Pregnancy outcome and fertility control in Aberdeen', *British Journal of Preventive and Social Medicine*, 27: 137–45.

Thompson, B and Baird, D (1967), 'Some impressions of childbearing in tropical areas', Parts I, II and III. *Journal of Obstetrics and Gynaecology of British Commonwealth*, 74: 329–38; 499–522.

Thompson, B and Illsley, R (1969), 'Family growth in Aberdeen', *Journal of Biosocial Science*, 1: 23–9.

Thompson, B, Illsley, R and Halliwell, R (1984), 'Psychosocial aspects of VTP in historical perspective: a case study of North-East Scotland'. In: *Voluntary termination of pregnancy* (ed) Hafez, E S E (MTP Press Ltd, Lancaster).

Thomson, A M (1958), 'Diet in pregnancy. I. A dietary survey technique and the nutritive value of diet as taken by primigravidae', *British Journal of Nutrition*, 12: 446–61.

——(1959a), 'Diet in pregnancy. II. Assessment of the nutritive value of diets, especially in relation to differences between Social classes', *British Journal of Nutrition*, 13: 190–204.

——(1959b), 'Diet in pregnancy. III. Diet in relation to the course and outcome of pregnancy', *British Journal of Nutrition*, 13: 509–25.

Titmuss, R (1943), *Birth, poverty and wealth* (Hamish Hamilton, London).

Walker, J and Turnbull, E P N (1953), 'Haemoglobin and red cells in human foetus and their relation to oxygen content of blood vessels of umbilical cord', *Lancet*, ii: 312–18.

Young, M and Willmott, P (1957) *Family and Kinship in East London* (Routledge and Kegan Paul, London).

Author Index

Subject Index